How to get

PAID

for what you've earned

by John Wilson

Medical Economics Company
Oradell, New Jersey 07649

ISBN 0-87489-042-X

Medical Economics Company
Oradell, New Jersey 07649

First Printing   June, 1974
Second Printing September, 1975

Publisher's Notes

About the author:

This book of helpful, practical advice and suggestions for doctors and their assistants is the synthesis of John Wilson's 20 years of experience in medical and business administration. He is currently head of MD Business Office Consultants, Bandon-by-the-Sea, Oregon, and on the Advisory Board of Medicon Corporation's San Francisco-based medical service bureaus. As an authority on medical credit and collections, he has published many articles on the subject in professional magazines. He is also the author of "Teenager's Introduction to Credit," soon to be published in paperback.

Acknowledgments:

The author gratefully acknowledges the assistance of Patricia Parson of Credit Bureaus, Inc., and Leonard Sklar of Medicon Corporation, for their invaluable suggestions; attorneys Melvin Belli, George Gant, Al C. Walsh, and John Murray, for their patience in answering endless legal questions; William T. Metts, Ph.D., for providing an objective viewpoint; and the hundreds of insurance companies that supplied necessary information and matériel.

The publisher and editor are indebted to John C. Post, Professional Business Management, Inc., Washington, D.C., and H. David Whieldon, formerly senior associate editor of Medical Economics magazine, for their perceptive advice and counsel; and to Fred Witzig, Tenafly, New Jersey, who designed the book.

Table of Contents

1

Creating your office policy

"Three basic choices"

As the new patient enters your office he passes from his world into yours. At that moment he's open and receptive to the laws governing this new environment. But if it seems that there are none, he'll make his own. So it's up to you, as you welcome a new addition to your practice, to set the rules of the relationship.

Most people are impressed by efficiency. If your business office is running like the countdown for a space launching, it lends a feeling of confidence. Consider your own feelings when you try out a new restaurant. A slovenly waitress and a dirty table may conceal an excellent kitchen, but they'll certainly make you look twice at the soup, won't they? So for the sake of the patient, as well as yourself, you need to create a definite office policy and require that it be followed.

This chapter examines three basic types of office policy. Their differences arise mainly from differences in doctors' attitudes toward money-making. But since money is essential to civilized life, the differences are necessarily of degree rather than kind. It must be assumed that most physicians want all three of medicine's prime rewards: a good income, the satisfaction of service to humanity, and the exhilarating exercise of the beneficial power bestowed by medical science. Your own office disciplines, therefore, are likely to depend on what you want **most** from your practice. If you're uncertain about the relative degrees of your interest, the tables on the following page may be helpful.

Know yourself Your practice will run more smoothly and you'll better achieve your personal goals if you clearly decide in which direction you should face.

The little test below may clarify this for you.

Income Goal

I Financial	$40,000	$50,000	$60,000	$70,000	More

Emotional Involvement

II Humanitarian	Little	Some	Average	Much	Full

Intellectual Motivation

III Scientific	20%	40%	60%	80%	100%

	I	II	III
Your Formula			

Heavy on line I = Money-maker
Heavy on line II = Humanitarian
Heavy on line III = Scientist

Money-maker

If you believe that in addition to serving humanity you're entitled to a good living and a reasonable return on your years of training;

If you believe that when your patients stop paying your bills promptly it's time to change the way you're running your business, then the first section of this chapter can help you.

By taking what you can use from this book and by requiring your staff to follow the precepts you adapt to your own situation, you can "fine tune" your business office and turn losses into profits.

Humanitarian

If you became a doctor primarily because you need to help people;

If the financial end of your practice is just a necessary evil that allows you to continue with your real interest, which is working with people as a healer and friend;

And if forcing people to pay bills goes against your grain, then the second section is intended for you. It will allow you to run an efficient office without any sacrifice of your principles.

8

Scientist

You didn't spend all those years at medical school just to become a bookkeeper. In fact, you want nothing to do with the financial end of your practice. It doesn't interest you, and it tends to come between you and your practice of medicine.

On the other hand, you do expect to receive proper compensation for your work.

If you're willing, initially, to set your office up properly in a way that will keep it running smoothly, Section Three was designed for you.

Section One: Money-maker

Rule One: Adopt a really good patient registration form.

Don't be embarrassed if your form asks lots of questions. In most cases, this is really a credit application. Before you actually extend credit, sometimes for hundreds of dollars, take a tip from Big Business: Get all the information.

Don't worry about offending your patients. People these days are quite used to filling out forms if they want credit. Beware of the patient who objects to filling out your form. At the very least he's a complainer; at worst, he's a credit criminal with plans to beat you out of your bill.

The patient registration form on page 10 is considered a good one. Train your assistants to insist that it be completely filled out.

Check it out: Have your assistant call at least two of the phone numbers on it—the patient's employer to verify that he's employed and has the insurance coverage claimed, and the previous physician's office to learn his experience with the patient.

Don't fall into the trap of believing that you can't afford to have your assistant take the time to do this on every patient. You may be paying her $3 to $4 an hour. The calls shouldn't take more than 10 minutes, which amounts to less than 70¢ worth of her time. Your final bill for this patient may be $300 or more—not including all the time your assistant may spend later trying to collect the bill because you didn't allow her time to check the form out properly at the beginning.

In most cases, the calls will prove that the information given by the would-be patient is legitimate. But the times when you do catch a bad one are well worth the small investment.

Retain the form: If the account does go bad, your assistant should send a photocopy to the collection agency when she assigns the account. It will appreciably increase the agency's chances of making the collection.

Advance payment policy: Most patients have some sort of insurance. But the time to make sure is when the patient is on the phone asking

NAME (MISS or MRS)	BIRTH DATE	SEX	NAME OF SPOUSE

ADDRESS		TEL:

OCCUPATION	SS #	BUSINESS TELEPHONE

EMPLOYER	EMPLOYER ADDRESS

PERSON RESPONSIBLE FOR PAYMENT

NAME	RELATIONSHIP TO PATIENT	TEL:

ADDRESS	SS #

EMPLOYER	OCCUPATION	BUSINESS TELEPHONE

BANK INFORMATION—BRANCH   CHECKING   SAVINGS

EMPLOYER'S ADDRESS   DRIV. LICENSE

HOW WILL BILL BE PAID?

PREVIOUS DOCTOR:	DATE OF LAST TREATMENT

NEAREST RELATIVE IN AREA:	TEL:

ADDRESS:

WHO REFERRED YOU TO US?

INSURANCE CO.:	GROUP #	LOCAL #

INSURANCE NAME IF DIFFERENT FROM PATIENT:

HOW MUCH IS THE DEDUCTIBLE:	DID YOU BRING FORMS?

ACKNOWLEDGMENT & AUTHORITY

I consent to treatment as necessary or desirable to the care of the patient first named above, including but not restricted to whatever drugs, medicine, performance of operations and conduct of laboratory, x-ray, or other studies that may be used by the attending doctor, or his nurse or qualified designate.

I also acknowledge full responsibility for the payment of such services and agree to pay for them, in full, AT THE TIME OF SERVICE, unless other arrangements are made with the Financial Department.

Signed: PATIENT, PARENT, OR AGENT_____

MEDICAL INFORMATION

HIGH BLOOD PRESSURE	ANEMIA	EAR TROUBLE
HEART TROUBLE	KIDNEY OR LIVER PROBLEMS	TUBERCULOSIS
DIABETES	ARTHRITIS	
ASTHMA	EYE TROUBLE	ARE YOU PREGNANT?

WHEN WAS YOUR LAST VISIT TO A DENTIST?

ARE YOU SUBJECT TO PROFUSE BLEEDING?	ARE YOU ALLERGIC TO PENICILLIN OR NOVOCAINE?

All delinquencies are reported to MEDICON CORP.,
the service bureau available to all doctors,
clinics and hospitals in the Bay Area.

for that first appointment. Before deciding on a policy of asking for advance payments, check the experience of other doctors in the area.

In any event, during the first phone call, your assistant can use an advance payment request as a counterbalance to her request that the patient bring insurance claim forms with him. She can say: "Please be sure to bring your insurance claim forms with you. That way we can excuse you from the $20 advance fee required of new patients."

Rule Two: Lay it on the line.

Don't underestimate the value of stating your policies clearly to the patient. If you expect to have each appointment paid for prior to the next one, say so, preferably in writing. One way to do this is the brochure.

All you really need is a one- or two-page folder, envelope size, that states your advance policy, credit policy, policy on insurance forms, and pleasure in having the family as new patients.

It should be mailed after the initial phone call. It serves to reinforce the instructions your assistant gave over the phone. Also, keep a supply in plain view in your waiting room.

Your patients won't object to your rules, provided you give them plenty of advance warning. They certainly will resent being caught unprepared, or not having the opportunity to find another doctor if they don't like your policies.

They appreciate knowing where they stand. They wish to avoid embarrassment at all costs and they'll respect you, even if your credit policy is tough. Just be certain you're consistent and make clear from the start just what you expect.

Deductibles: Another loss leader that a little care can avoid is the annual deductible that most group policies include. The patient may not even realize that the deductible exists. Even if he says it's been met, you had better check it out with his previous doctor.

The indispensable assistant: Be sure to have short training sessions with your office staff. Let them know you're interested in how they're carrying out your policies.

Do put those policies in writing and see that each assistant has a copy.

Don't assume that your policies will continue indefinitely. They won't. You'll need to reinforce them from time to time as your assistants begin to slack off.

Do spot-check your delinquent accounts. Find out if the billing was done on time, and if the registration form was properly checked out. If your assistants consider you thorough, they'll be thorough, too.

Do hire an assistant who can be firm on the phone, but DON'T make the mistake of hiring a tiger. Harsh collection techniques are out of place in a doctor's office and cause many more problems than they solve.

You determine the office atmosphere. It should be warm and friendly, but strictly businesslike, with a pride taken in its efficiency.

You're also usually in the best position to discuss finances with the patient, particularly for future surgery or long-term therapy. You can give the best estimate of the cost and, in the course of the discussion, you can find out how the patient plans to handle it.

Rule Three: Stick to your office policy.

If you can't follow it yourself, your assistants will take the easy way out, too. Your best bet is not to offer long-term credit to anyone. Leave that to the banks or finance companies.

If your patient absolutely can't raise the money, you may want to suggest a state or county organization that can help, or you may decide to discount the bill. Either way, don't vacillate. Make a clear-cut decision both for yourself and for the patient.

Final credit tip: Don't hang on to delinquent accounts too long. The most serious single mistake that doctors make is to bill nonpaying accounts month after month, thus wasting staff time in nonproductive work. Never hold on to a delinquent account for more than six months. In fact, four months is a better deadline if you receive absolutely no payment. Get them off your list of concerns and let an agency worry about them. Remember, you pay an agency nothing unless it collects.

Section Two: Humanitarian

Rule One: Have a brochure stating your policy regarding payment of bills. If some of your patients get the idea that you are too easy they will take advantage of you.

An inoffensive but effective brochure used by one doctor reads:

> "Dear Patient:
>
> All I'm interested in is your health. The bill I will send you pays for the cost of running this office and helps support my family, but it isn't the reason that I became a doctor.
>
> It will help if you will pay for each visit as you leave, but if you can't, you will be sent a bill. When you receive it, please call the nurse and tell her how you will pay it. If you need time, she will give it to you.
>
> In any event, don't let the bill deter you from seeking my help whenever you need it.
>
> Your doctor"

Each new patient is handed the brochure along with a short registration form that merely asks for name, address, phone number, patient's or spouse's place of employment, and pertinent insurance information.

Rule Two: To make up for losses in other areas, and to prevent a lack of funds from forcing you to adopt a tougher attitude toward your patients, you'll want to collect every penny you can from insurance companies. So be sure your assistant is well versed in insurance billing.

Some insurance companies, the "Blues" in particular, will often send a representative to instruct your assistant. However, here's another tip that can pay off: Check with the insurance department of your local hospital. The insurance clerk there is usually an expert. She can give your assistant many valuable tips and will remain available for free advice because she'll tend to regard your assistant as a sort of protégée.

Rule Three: Indoctrinate your staff. Talk to them long and fairly often about your philosophy. If you have an open dissenter whom you can't convert, get rid of her; otherwise she'll put pressure on patients behind your back. Many people have what amounts to absolute ideas of right and wrong, and they're not likely to let patients get away with anything just because you're a "softy."

Rule Four: Don't use a collection agency. Reason: You can't control their actions after you've assigned accounts to them.

The agency's salesman, when he visits your office, seems to be a great guy who agrees with your policies wholeheartedly—but he's not the one who'll be hounding your patients. Your admirable philosophy of "humanity first" is not generally shared by professional collectors. Their job is to get the money, and they'll do whatever is necessary, within the law, to get it for you.

Section Three: Scientist

Rule One: Think of your office as a machine. You've got to start the motor and get it running right before you can turn your back on it. And you've got to return from time to time to tune it up again.

So get yourself the best office manager you can find and pay well enough to keep her. But don't get a tiger. If you do, you'll find your practice thinning out fast. They may like you, but patients will feel that getting by the dragon at the gate is more trouble than your healing talents are worth.

Rule Two: Use a good, comprehensive patient registration form such as the one illustrated earlier (see page 10). Always have it checked out.

An outside computerized billing service and an outside bookkeeping service make sense for you, because they'll eliminate two areas that might otherwise distract you. If you practice in a small community and the billing service is not locally available, don't hesitate to contact one outside your area. Distance seems to make little or no difference in their relative efficiency. A word of caution:

If you do use an outside billing service, require it to return your accounts instead of automatically assigning them to a collection agency after their normal billing cycle is completed. Collection agencies aren't equally effective, and you'll want to choose the best.

Rule Three: Leave selection of a collection agency to your office manager. If she's holding the bag for this she'll be inclined to demand good results from them. Also, it will relieve you of having to talk to their representatives.

But be sure to have the accounts go through a "free letter" service first. Most agencies make this service available, as a sales device, but you may have to ask for it. Usually the process, which gives fair warning to patients, involves one, two, or three letters sent by the agency in its name asking the patient to pay you directly, **before** the account is assigned for collection.

Such letters usually collect about 20 per cent of the accounts you list. The rest are retained by the agency and listed for collection. A free letter service, as the name implies, costs you nothing. But the agency will expect you to assign to them all those who don't pay for regular collection procedures.

Rule Four: Establish a definite office policy. And make clear to office personnel that it can't be changed without your approval. That makes it official, and your office manager and assistants can have confidence in it and use the necessary firmness to carry it out.

Once you have an office policy established and running smoothly, don't involve yourself in a patient's financial problems. Turn over all requests about the cost of your services or manner of payment to your office manager, and let her decision be final. In other words, don't meddle.

Just make sure that your patients learn of the policy at the time they register. A brochure, described in Section One, is a good method which leaves little room for misunderstanding.

Finally, even though you're anxious to stay away from the financial end, do spot-check from time to time. Have an occasional policy meeting with your manager. There will always be some problems that require your personal intervention, but by setting your office up in this way you'll eliminate a myriad of petty details.

2

Getting the most out of your billing

"Meeting a monthly deadline"

A great part of your revenue these days undoubtedly comes from your third-party billing. The proportion may vary from office to office but it certainly adds up to a significant share of your income. But what about the remainder?

Curiously, the remainder seldom gets the attention and professional handling that it should, even though it may be 20 per cent of your total revenue and involve, through balances due after insurance payments, at least 80 per cent of your patients.

In most offices the billing of patients is done once a month. It's a time of tension and disruption. And as a necessary but tiresome chore, it's done in an automatic and mechanical way, and finished as quickly as possible. If you couple this unimaginative procedure with the fact that most debtors place their medical bills at the end of the line in order of urgency, you wonder that any doctor ever gets paid.

That you do collect most of your money, eventually, underlines the general belief that most people are basically honest. However, you can collect more money, more quickly, and at less expense by using better billing techniques.

Billing a huge receivable in a large clinic and individually handling a few accounts in a solo doctor's limited practice are hardly comparable, and we'll be proposing a different procedure for each. Nevertheless, there are several universal constants that apply to both.

For best results, any billing should be prompt, accurate, and effective. By prompt, I mean setting and meeting a billing deadline each month.

Billing that is not accurate results in endless extra work as you call or write back and forth, and may even provoke the patient into not paying at all.

Effective billing results in payment. Routinely sending out identical statements, month after month, is the least effective and most expensive way to collect your accounts.

Delay is your enemy. Each patient should get your bill while the service is fresh in his mind, and while he still has the money to pay it. As time passes, other bills of all kinds eat away at his budget, and the urgency to pay you fades under the clamor of more recent creditors. So if you want your money, you must motivate patients to pay you now, not get worked up about it 90 days from now. And the more closely your billing is tailored to the individual patient, the better your chances of being paid promptly.

One doctor I know has a very smooth and practical routine. After the initial visit for X-rays and examination, he discusses the patient's needs and the cost of the work to be done. A program of visits is worked out, and then the patient is introduced to the office manager.

The manager offers a program of monthly payments, complete with payment book, and requests that a reasonably small down payment be brought to the next appointment. Without any sparring back and forth, the agreement is made for payment. The payment dates and amounts are tailored to fit the patient's budget. Gone is the usual apprehension that a patient feels about how much all this will cost him, or how he is going to raise the money when the doctor gets through. Everything is settled in advance.

Critics of this system might argue that under it you could find yourself giving credit when, in some cases at least, you didn't need to. I disagree. Most people who can afford to pay their bills promptly and in full don't want to bother with monthly payments. On the other hand, it provides the great advantage of prompting less affluent patients who haven't done so to think seriously about how they're going to pay.

That may not be your way. It may not even be applicable in your practice. But the lesson that may be learned from it is that **you**, rather than the patient, should set the rules for extending credit, and as early as possible in the relationship.

In a small office, a dynamic and highly personalized approach can be made to the problem of billing. The first step is to discard the inflexible, once a month system of billing patients. Your billing system should be designed to:

— promptly determine the reason for nonpayment,

- make close and exact follow-ups of payment plans, and
- include an effective method of motivating payment.

Let's take each of those points in order:

What you don't want is your assistant rebilling a patient, month after month, without giving you enough information to decide whether to write off the account or assign it to an agency. That's expensive in terms of supplies, postage, and your staff's time. Also, as the account gets older, it becomes progressively less collectible. For that reason, if you don't get paid after the first statement, you need to find out why. You can't assume that the patient is just a little short this month and that you'll probably receive payment next month. Your assistant's questioning may be the factor that actually motivates payment. It also lets you know if the reason for nonpayment is some dissatisfaction with your treatment.

The best way to get such information is on the phone. That way, your assistant can adjust her questions to the reaction of the patient. But if a phone call isn't practical, I suggest sending the following form letter in place of your next statement:

> Dear Mr.
>
> Dr. Jones has asked me to send you a note to find out why your balance of $_____ still due on your account has not been paid.
>
> If the reason has been a temporary shortage of funds, please don't feel embarrassed to call me and explain. This can happen to anyone, and I will be most happy to work something out with you.
>
> I need to hear from you right away because our C.P.A. is coming on Friday and I have to go over our past-due accounts with him. I just don't want yours to be included and if we can work something out, it won't.
>
> Here is my number:_____ Please call me.
>
> Sincerely,
>
> Mrs. _____
> Bookkeeper for Dr. Jones

You can have a perfect copy of this letter typed and sent to the printer with a ream of your letterhead paper for inexpensive reproduction as a form letter. Your assistant can then type in name, address, date, and amount due as required.

You can accomplish a close and exact follow-up of patient payments without great additional work for your assistant by having more than one alphabetical breakdown of your receivables. Ideally, you may decide to have three:

Group 1 — Patients on payment plans.

Group 2 — Patients on your "Hot File."

Group 3 — Other patients.

Group 1 are those patients who have agreed to pay off their accounts over several or many monthly payments. Keep them in a separate file. At the time arrangements are made, the patient's ledger is tagged with a date three days before his monthly payment is due:

```
                                               ┌──────┐
                                               │  21  │
┌──────────────────────────────────────────────┴──────┴──┐
│                                                         │
│     Patient:   George Jones                             │
 \___/_____/_____/_____/_____/\____/\__/
```

Once each day, your assistant flips through these accounts and sends out a reminder envelope on those with today's date. This statement includes the balance due, a receipt for last month's payment, and a line explaining that the plan may continue only as long as the payments remain prompt and regular.

Since the patient set up these arrangements for a time in the month most convenient for making a payment, your reminder will arrive at exactly the right time. Thus, your chances of being included in the bills he pays this month are greatly improved.

You've done your part, but getting the reminder to the patient at the right time will still not always get your money. You need some follow-up device to signal you if the payment is not made.

The surest way is to use a payment record. This can be a simple loose-leaf book containing 31 numbered pages, one for every day of the month.

When a patient arranges to make his payment on a certain day, say the 15th, his name is entered on page 15 of the payment record. When your assistant checks the payment record each day and sees that payment hasn't been received on the date promised, she sends out the "late payment" notice (see illustration), or she calls the patient. The point is, you **cultivate** these payment plans. Patients under financial pressures will put off paying those creditors who don't appear too anxious about their money. Doctors are generally at the end of the line.

It's not hard to put yourself at the head, though, if you put a reminder in the patient's hands at the right time of the month, follow up to see that the payment is made, and always contact the patient immediately when payment is either late or not made.

All this may seem like a lot of extra work for your assistant, but it really isn't. The hidden advantage is that the more precisely and

Advance notice statement for payment plans

Mr. George Jones
941 Stateline Boulevard
San Francisco, California 94104

Your last payment received: _____ $
Balance now: $
Your next payment due the 24th.

As we agreed, continuation of this payment
program depends on promptness and regularity.
Please send your payment today.

Thank you.

The reverse side of the flap bears the doctor's name,
address, and prepaid postage imprint.

Late payment notice

Mr. George Jones
941 Stateline Blvd.
San Francisco, Ca. 94104

LATE PAYMENT REMINDER

Your payment was not received on the date agreed
upon. As you know, our C.P.A. will require us to
discontinue the arrangement if payment is not received
as agreed.

If you send payment today in this envelope we will
reinstate your plan, otherwise please make arrangements
to have the balance in full on your account in this office
within seven days.

Thank you.

efficiently she does it, the less need you'll have for the follow-up. Your patients quickly become educated to your system and save their games for other, more lax creditors.

Here's a tip if you have more than one assistant. Place the responsibility for the follow-up squarely on the shoulders of one. Then, once in a while, leaf through the file to see how she's doing.

The second alphabet in your system is the Hot File. These are patients who have made no financial arrangements with you. They're receiving your statements and ignoring them. They didn't respond to the letter your assistant sent to determine their status. Your assistant can't reach them by phone or gets nowhere with them when she does.

These are the accounts that require a decision from you, and the longer you wait, the less collectible they become.

Usually this isn't a very large file, so a great deal of money isn't involved. But it's a leak in the system and some of your income is running through it, so why not do something about it? Should you just write the accounts off? Should you assign them to a collection agency?

There are several steps you can take. The first is to get the attention of the patient who up until now has not taken you very seriously. In our training classes for collectors we often hear the plaintive question: "What if I can't reach the debtor on the phone and I send every notice we have and he still doesn't respond? What am I supposed to do?" We call it: The case of the impervious debtor.

It's quite common in units operated by inexperienced collectors, though it becomes quite rare as they mature. The more experienced collector insists on getting and holding the attention of the debtor.

The question is: How? The best way is to get him on the telephone (covered in the next chapter). Failing that, try one of these:

Step 1: A note requesting that he call your office today sent to his place of employment in a plain envelope marked **personal.** Why on the job? To cover the possibility that his wife is just not showing him your bills, and because he probably won't want letters coming to him at work and will contact you to prevent its happening again.

Step 2: A plain postcard, handwritten, addressed to his wife, asking her to call you without delay and giving the office number. Have your assistant sign it.

Step 3: A night letter (an inexpensive telegram) sent to his home, asking him to call you at the office.

Allow two days between steps for him to answer. Don't mention your bill on any of them, and there's an almost 100 per cent chance that by the third notice, he or his wife will have contacted you.

When your assistant gets either one on the phone, she should mince no words: Failure to pay, she tells them, requires that she assign the account to an agency for collection. She doesn't want this to happen and

STEP 1: NOTE c/o EMPLOYMENT

Dear Mr. Jones:

     Please call me sometime today. It is quite important that I speak to you.

     My number is: _____

                Dr. Brown

STEP 2: POSTCARD

Dear Mrs. Jones,

Very important that you call me. Today

843-2100

Pat Clark

Dr. Brown's Office

STEP 3: TELEGRAM

URGENT THAT YOU CALL MY OFFICE TODAY

MY NUMBER IS _____

THIS IS IMPORTANT TO YOU

DR. BROWN

that's why she made such an effort to get in touch.

A logical follow-up, if they ignore your efforts, is to use the precollection service provided by your collection agency. If that doesn't work, your best bet is to assign the account without further delay. The use of the Hot File accomplishes this for you:

1. It brings to the surface your bad accounts very early in the game.
2. It's reassurance that you're doing everything possible to get the accounts to pay.
3. It gives your patient every opportunity to discuss his problems with you and ensures that he won't be taken by surprise if you have to assign the account to an agency.

Usually, when he contacts you, he will arrange for payments of some sort. This is the time to transfer his account from the Hot File into your payment plan file. Insist on some phone numbers where you can reach him in the future. It can save you a lot of trouble.

If your operation is too large, or your system too complex to use the three-file system, you can still step up the efficiency and effectiveness of your billings in other ways.

I've had experience with large groups whose monthly write-off and assignment to me was enough to support a small agency. This was great business for me because it was so easily collectible. The patients had received no more pressure than a series of identical statements. The shock to them, when they were assigned to me, was enough to collect the bills without any further effort on my part.

It's really necessary that accounts have some sort of personalized, "tailored-to-the-specific-case" collection activity before you write them off. Otherwise you're throwing money away. A limited effort in this direction can be made by enclosing a statement of your credit policy with the first notice you send out.

You can also change the color of your statements from month to month and thus winnow new accounts from old. For example: If the second statement is yellow, and you use window envelopes, you can hold up mailing them until a call has been made and the reason for nonpayment ascertained. With the third statement, which might be blue, you can enclose another form letter. (See example B.) Switch to a windowless envelope for the third notice to give it the best possible chance of being opened. Then, on the 15th, if no money has been received and the patient hasn't contacted you to make satisfactory arrangements, assign the account to your agency for their precollection letter service.

This free service has several advantages: It usually gives the patient two more opportunities to pay you directly. You incur no fee from the agency. And the patient is not officially assigned for collection. But if the letters are also ignored, you can feel fairly sure that nothing you

Statement of credit policy "A"

Dear Patient:

We have had many requests to put our credit policy in writing. Everyone likes to know where he or she stands financially, and so we are including this letter with your statement.

INSURANCE

If you have insurance and bring us your claim form, we will complete and forward it for you at no charge.

If you assign your benefits to us, we will allow you credit for the amount we estimate insurance will pay. The balance will be billed to you and we will require that you pay it now, while we are waiting for the insurance to pay.

If the insurance should either reject your claim or pay less than we calculated, we will then bill you for the difference.

MONTHLY STATEMENTS

All statements are due and payable in full when you receive them, unless prior arrangements have been made.

If the bill remains unpaid, with no satisfactory arrangements, then, on the advice of our C.P.A., the account will be assigned to a collection agency.

The credit manager is Mrs. Jeffrey. Any credit arrangements must be made with her.

The Clinic, like any other business organization, depends upon its income to keep operating. Your assistance will be most appreciated.

Very truly yours,

Business Manager

> **Statement of credit policy "B"**
>
> Dear Patient:
>
> As we explained to you earlier, our financial policy as set
> by our C.P.A. requires that all bills be paid promptly.
>   Your bill is now 90 days past due and unless we receive
> payment from you by the 15th it will automatically be
> assigned to an agency for collection.
>   If you want to avoid this action, we suggest that you
> put your check in the mail today.
>
>   Very truly yours,
>
>   Credit Manager

could have done would have prompted the patient to pay, and that it's
time for the professional collectors to take over.

    Having a firm credit policy and assigning your accounts at the right
time puts you in a much sounder financial position than a clinic that
carries huge accounts receivable, extending over many months. As time
passes, much of what they're carrying becomes uncollectible, even by an
agency, and the burden of billing and rebilling remains expensive, time-
consuming, and unprofitable. Moreover, a clearly spelled-out credit policy
gradually becomes public knowledge. You'll find more of your bills
being paid promptly because the patients know exactly where they stand.

3

Collecting by telephone

"A sense of urgency"

> WANTED: Telephone Collector. Must be tough
> and hard-hitting. Gravel voice an asset.
> Sob sisters need not apply. Write Box 86.

Anyone who answered an ad like that would be bad news in a doctor's office. In fact, she'd be more liability than asset, even in a hard-line commercial credit office.

Granted, the purpose of a phone call is to collect money. But that goal must be achieved with finesse. The debtor must be allowed to save face; the doctor's image must be maintained—even enhanced—by the call. And the way must be left open for follow-up calls, where necessary. So the ad should read:

> WANTED: Doctor's assistant. A sympathetic but
> practical person; pleasant-voiced, but positive;
> to interview patients by telephone. Box 86.

Experience has shown that a skilled telephone collector working in your office can get money for you faster (thus saving most of those collection agency fees) and still save debtors as patients. More important: By conducting a dialogue with patients, she may even save you from an expensive malpractice suit.

Best of all, it may not even be necessary to hire a girl to make these calls. Your present assistant, if she has the time and aptitude, can do it for you. Just bear in mind that something more practical than a pat on the head should be her reward if she does the job enthusiastically and successfully.

The rest of this chapter contains explicit instructions and examples for your employe to follow. Have her read it, then turn her loose and let her try. Before you do, however, make an "aging" analysis of your accounts receivable by months. That will give you the dollar value owed in consecutive 30-day periods. By comparing each month against the previous one, you'll be able to judge the progress being made in keeping your accounts more current.

Instructions for a beginning telephone collector

So you're going to be a telephone collector and add one more skill to your portfolio. Well, don't be afraid. And if you are, don't show it. The only time you'll have trouble with normal debtors on the phone is when they sense that you're afraid of them. (Neophyte lion tamers probably get this same advice, too.)

To be a successful collector, you must concentrate on projecting your emotions through the telephone. Almost everyone knows how. You've done it many times yourself, talking to your husband, friends, or your folks. But for some reason, when a business call is involved, people tend to bottle up their emotions and let very little seep through. That doesn't mean you need to rant, rave, or bully. But you will have to reason, persuade, and convince people to do what you ask. You can't do it by talking in a flat, businesslike way, completely devoid of emotion. You've got to be warm, concerned, and, most of all, enthusiastic.

People react in a mirrorlike way to emotion. If you're angry, they get angry. If you're friendly, they're friendly. And if you conjure up a sense of urgency, they'll feel a similar urgency.

By developing your technique, you'll soon learn to engage their emotions in a direct, vibrant, and very positive way. To do a good job, you should know the **why, when,** and **how** of telephone collecting. Let's start by looking at the typical patient and his attitude:

Every month he's dealt a fistful of bills. Yours is just one among them. So why should he pay you first? After all, if he doesn't pay the finance company they'll come and take his car. But the doctor's bill? Why bother? His attitude will be completely different, however, if you've called him. Being a good telephone collector, you extracted his promise to pay. Besides, you were nice to him and he's going to feel a twinge of guilt if he overlooks you. Someone else will just have to wait.

MEMO: Objectives in collecting by telephone
1. To create a sense of urgency about payment.
2. To keep payment plans prompt.

3. To prevent overdue accounts from going to a collection agency.
   As you can see, if you reach those objectives, it will have a direct influence on your doctor's income.

MEMO: Why telephone collecting is effective
1. A telephone call is difficult to ignore. Slow-paying patients can throw your notices away without reading them, but they can never ignore you when you call.
2. You can tailor the call to fit the patient. A call can be stepped up or eased off as conversation continues, something you can't do in a written notice.
3. You can extract a commitment to pay. Patients have to react to your call. And if you've been persuasive, they find they've promised to pay you.

MEMO: Dangers in collecting by telephone
1. If you're unprepared, you may find yourself outtalked.
2. If you can be drawn into a quarrel, you may provide the excuse the patient needs for nonpayment of the bill.
   Both of those dangers are very real. If you get off on the wrong foot, or don't have all your facts straight, you'll be in trouble. In some cases, if the debtor seizes this advantage and uses it to rattle you, he may be able to make you angry and force a quarrel. That gives him a dandy reason for delaying payment.

MEMO: Advantages in collecting by telephone
1. *Speed.* You can call today and find the money in the mail tomorrow.
2. *Gripes.* Resentments, real or imagined, that might result in a lost patient, or even a malpractice suit, surface and can be dealt with.
3. *Cash.* You not only get money in faster, you get more of it. A patient who planned to send only a nominal payment can be persuaded to send the entire balance.
4. *Frustration.* You avoid the frustration of billing month after month and not getting even the courtesy of a reply. Decisive action, which you can take right now on the phone, is a great antidote to that feeling of helplessness.

Now that you know **why** there's need to make telephone collection calls, let's look at the **when** and **how**:

Make the call two weeks after sending the second statement; or two weeks after the last billing, if it's a continuing billing on a longtime patient. That schedule gives the patient a reasonable time to send his check, and saves you unnecessary calls. But when the time comes to call, be sure to use collection agencies' secret weapon—persistence. If the patient isn't home, or puts you off, **always** call back.

In the pages to come, you'll be getting plenty of examples of what to say when you call. But first read through this list of five dos and don'ts:

1. *Don't attack.* Once you do, you've raised a barrier between you and the patient. You're no longer communicating.

2. *Don't prejudge.* Never imply criticism of any kind. A negative approach will reap only a negative response.

3. *Do reassure.* Let the patient know you have a good opinion of him. You might say something along this line: "I know you'd never have let this bill go without a very good reason."

4. *Do listen.* And sympathize, even if briefly.

5. *Do explain.* Tell why the bill must be paid now, remembering that your reason must be valid from the patient's point of view. So don't expect payment if the reason you give is that the doctor wants his money. Instead, try one of these approaches:

— "Our accountant is coming in this week and I don't want him to see that **your** account is not paid."

— "You know, your **good medical credit** is a very real asset, especially when **you or your family get sick.**"

— "You're responsible for this account, and I've already allowed more time than I should. How can I explain to the doctor that you haven't paid?"

Your first phone call

Before picking up the phone, analyze the account. Decide on a minimum acceptable amount if you can't persuade the patient to pay in full. Ask yourself if there's anything unusual about the account. Is the patient the mayor's mother-in-law? A widow with four children? A little old lady with a bad heart? An unemployed father? In other words, is there anything about the patient's status that requires unusually delicate handling?

If not, and you have more than one phone number, decide which to call first. Avoid calling a patient at work with the first call. Later, if he still fails to pay, by all means reach him there.

If the only number you have is that of a relative, neighbor, or friend, don't reveal the purpose of your call. It might cause your patient embarrassment. Don't mention the bill at all. Just say: "Would you please have Mrs. Jones call Nancy at Dr. Smith's office?"

Use the call to verify information about the patient. Find out, for example, if his wife is working. Anything you learn may prove valuable later, should the account become a true delinquent.

Aim to end the conversation with **you** in control. Don't allow the patient to make a speech and then hang up on you. Interrupt, if necessary. If you feel that the call is becoming too drawn out, or if the patient tries to get you off the phone, say:

"I'm sorry, Mr. Gordon, but I have other patients waiting so I'm going to have to say good-by. Before I do, though, I've noted on your chart that you'll be mailing the check today, so we should have it by Wednesday at the latest. Thank you very much. Good-by."

Or, if the call hasn't been successful:

"Well, Mr. Gordon, do please talk this over with your wife when she comes home. I must get this cleared up, one way or another, before our C.P.A. shows up this week. I'll call you back tomorrow. Thank you. Good-by."

If that's inappropriate, try this:

"I'm sorry to hear you say that, Mr. Gordon. Just remember, though, if you change your mind, the C.P.A. won't be here until Friday. Be sure to call me before then. Thanks. Good-by."

Now you're ready for your first collection call. You've glanced at the patient's folder. You have his bill in front of you, along with a pencil and pad. You know what his balance is, how long it has been unpaid, and what is the smallest amount you'll settle for. The call may go like this:

"Hello, Mrs. Jones? This is Nancy at Dr. Smith's office. How are you this morning?"

"Oh, I'm fine thanks, and yourself?"

"Fine, thank you, but very busy. We're going through the accounts today, and we've noticed that we haven't received your check yet. Do you have a question about the bill that I could help you with?"

"Well, no. No question. It's just that we haven't had the money to pay it off all at once. I'm not back to work yet, you know."

"I see. Do you expect to return soon?"

"Oh, I should be going back on Monday, if all goes well. Then we plan on paying the doctor so much a month from my paycheck, if that's all right."

"Well, that sounds very good, Mrs. Jones, with everything under control. Now, let's see . . . I'll just note down here, for the doctor when he goes through the accounts, the date on which we can expect your payment. He likes me to do that on each account. Today is the 10th. May I put down that you'll clear the balance by the 30th?"

"Well, I'm not sure that I can do it by the 30th . . . let me see . . ."

"Perhaps I can help you, Mrs. Jones. When is your first payday? Next Friday, or is it every two weeks?"

"It's every two weeks."

"Well, in that case, suppose we say by the 12th of next month. That will give you two paydays. There, is that better?"

"Yes. I think I can do that."

"O.K., then, I'll put down that you'll pay half on the 29th, and the other half on the 12th. It's always best to get these things settled, don't you think, Mrs. Jones, rather than sending a bunch of notices back and forth? I'm so glad I called you. Keep well, and we'll look forward to seeing you when you come in for your checkup. Thanks again, Mrs. Jones. Good-by!"

Now, had Nancy not made that call, there's a good chance that Mrs. Jones would have procrastinated and not made a payment from her first paycheck. And almost certainly, the payment—if she did make it—wouldn't have been for half the bill. She might have sent $25, but more likely only $10.

Remember, your voice tone is almost as important as the words you say. Keep your voice friendly, cheerful, and energetic. Your patient, usually having lots of other bills to pay, may be depressed, lack confidence, feel hopeless. Be careful that your call doesn't reinforce those feelings. Instead, concentrate on uplifting her, inspiring her to do something about the bill, letting her sense that you're confident she can handle things properly.

Your call should be designed to motivate. In Nancy's call, because it was a first call, and because she didn't run into any real difficulties, the need to motivate was low. Mrs. Jones was told that the doctor went through the unpaid accounts and that he liked to see exactly when they would be cleared up. Nancy also mentioned that she would look forward to seeing Mrs. Jones at her next checkup, which implied that Mrs. Jones was still welcome, even though the bill was not yet paid.

Mrs. Jones, then, although behind in her bill, could still keep the doctor happy and stay in his good graces by keeping the payment arrangement Nancy had laid out for her. In other words, she was gently motivated to pay. If she fails to keep the arrangement, a follow-up call is in order. Of necessity, such calls have to be firmer and more to the point than your initial call, so it pays to have "motivating statements" ready. They're very useful when a patient has stumped you for words, or when you want to get the conversation back to the subject of payment. Here are eight of them:

1. I'd love to let you off your payment this month, but our C.P.A. has made a strict rule: If the payment isn't made, the payment plan is canceled. I'm very sorry.
2. Have you written the check for the doctor yet?
3. I have to go over the accounts with the doctor on Friday. I would like to have your check posted before then.
4. In order to keep your account on a current basis, we'll need to have your check in the office, ready to post, before Friday.
5. We refer all our overdue accounts to our C.P.A. on a monthly basis. Your check is overdue. Can you mail it today, or will you bring it in?
6. If the account remains unpaid, it will be referred to a collection

agency. If you don't want this to happen, you must mail your check in right away.

7. The collection agency picks up all delinquent accounts this Friday. I know you don't want yours included. Can you send someone in with the check today?
8. Your account has been referred to our bookkeeper for transfer to the collection agency. If you could bring in your check today, I could call her and stop it from going.

Type out this list and keep it in a permanent place, close to your phone, because you never know when a patient will call and say: "Gee, Nancy. I just can't make that payment I promised. Do me a favor and skip over me this month, will you?"

The first motivating phrase would allow you to answer this question without having the patient feel any animosity towards you.

Your second call will undoubtedly bring out a parade of excuses, stalls, and objections. It's all too easy to just accept the patient's "No" at face value and put the account aside for this month. If you do this, you will only have compounded the problem and made it more difficult for yourself when you call again next month. Whether he has a legitimate excuse, is just stalling, or has a genuine objection, you must deal with him **now.** You must recognize the difference:

— An **excuse** is a legitimate reason for not paying the bill: "My husband has been off work, as you know, with this injury and we didn't receive our first disability check until just this week. We paid the rent with that and will have to start paying you next month."
— A **stall** is a device to get you off the phone and buy more time for the debtor: "Oh, you'll have to talk to my husband about that; he takes care of all the bills. I don't know anything about it."
— An **objection** is nonpayment because of some fault—real or imagined—that the patient feels has been done him. Handled properly, an objection can be settled easily and the patient placated. However, mistaking this for a stall will really cause trouble for you and the doctor. "Yes, I'll be happy to tell you why I haven't paid the bill. You've got me down for an X-ray and I was never given an X-ray. Maybe I was supposed to get one and didn't, or maybe you're just charging me for something I didn't get. I don't know, but I'm not paying until you get it straight."

Here are common excuses and stalls and some workable responses to them:

Excuse: *"We just don't have the money. Things are very tight now."*
Response: "I know what you mean, but to keep your account on a

current basis we will need to receive your check for at least part of it this week."

Excuse: *"My husband's been unemployed. That's why we haven't been able to pay."*

Response: "That a shame but I'm glad to hear he's back to work now. I'll be talking to the doctor about these accounts this week. When can I tell him you will begin payments?"

Excuse: *"We thought the insurance would pay this."*

Response: "Very few insurances pay all of anyone's bill, but they did help you a lot with it. Now the rest is yours to pay. In order to keep your account on a current basis, I'll need to have your check in the office before Friday."

Excuse: *"Our attorney advised us not to pay any bills until our case is completely settled."*

Response: "Well, I think you should start making payments on the account because it's sometimes years before those things are settled, and it wouldn't be fair to the doctor to make him wait that long.

Stall: *"I mailed you the check for that last week."*

Response: "Well, since it hasn't arrived, we must assume that it was lost in the mail. Please send me another today and call your bank and stop payment on the first check. I'll call you tomorrow, when I receive your second check."

Stall: *"Mail me a statement and I'll be happy to send you a check."*

Response: "We've already mailed you several statements. Our C.P.A. requires that all accounts be kept on a current basis. You will need to get your check in the mail this afternoon. Can I tell him that you will?"

Stall: *"The insurance company should have paid more than they did. I don't want to pay on this bill until I get it cleared up with them."*

Response: "Really, this is a matter between the insurance company and you, although, of course, we'll be glad to help you with any information they need. Meanwhile, I need to receive your check before Friday, when I have to go over the accounts with the doctor."

Stall: *"I was planning to pay the whole bill from my income tax refund when it comes."*

Response: "We've already waited quite awhile for payment and now we have to show payment on the account or our C.P.A. will pick it up as a delinquent. We must have a check from you this week."

Whether it's an excuse or a stall, don't become inflexible. If the patient absolutely can't send full payment this week, settle for half. But use good judgment. Don't give in too easily, and don't settle for tiny payments. If you do, you'll be working on his account every month, for months to come.

On larger bills, offer suggestions and encouragement: "Have you considered trying to borrow the money, Mr. Smith?" Often, it will be up to you to instill enough confidence in him so that he will go out and try. Tell him that everyone has large medical bills at some time in his life, that banks and finance companies know this and are sympathetic, that they'll usually make special concessions, and that he'll be treated with courtesy and understanding. Besides, this might be a good opportunity for him to clear up all his other bills, too, so that he ends up with just one payment to make each month.

Objections constitute a special category—one in which you can be most valuable to your doctor. This is where your judgment, prompt action, and ability to satisfy not only can prevent patients from leaving your doctor, but may save him from an expensive lawsuit. If a patient's objection has anything to do with treatment, any careless or rough handling of his complaint could easily lead to a malpractice suit.

In handling objections, telephone contact has it all over sending out statements. You can send statements to an unhappy patient for months and end up referring the account to a collection agency without the patient ever telling you what was wrong. Then, before you know it, an attorney is in the picture, and no amount of talking will change that.

One properly made telephone call can avoid such headaches and probably save enough money to take care of all your delinquent accounts. So, when faced with an objection, question the patient carefully and politely. Take down all the information you can. Promise that you'll look into the matter personally, and that you'll call back just as soon as you have the answer. And be sure to do it!

In any case where the objection has to do with treatment, rather than billing, take it up with the doctor. Show him all your notes.

If it has to do with the bill, go over the ledger carefully. An extra five minutes here can save you a lot of time arguing with the patient and trying to collect later. If there's something he doesn't understand, explain fully and patiently until he does. Usually that's all it takes. Once satisfied that he isn't being ignored, the patient is happy to pay you.

Telephone collecting, like any other skill, has its shortcuts and techniques that have gradually developed through years of experience and thousands of calls. Failure in telephone collecting, perhaps more than in most things, tends to sap your self-confidence. Success, on the other hand, reinforces it. Here are 10 important rules to help you make successful follow-up calls:

1. Always use a third party when insisting on payment. (This may be your C.P.A., bookkeeper, or the doctor.)

2. Never accept an obvious stall.
3. Continually bring the conversation back to the subject of payment.
4. Keep the deadline for payment short. If you allow too much time, other creditors will contact your patient in between, and you won't get paid.
5. Inject a sense of urgency. This is done through your tone, what you say, and the short deadline.
6. Always have the last word. Leave the debtor with the message.
7. Keep the call short. If you talk too much, the message will be lost.
8. Don't be embarrassed to ask questions. You have the right to know anything that will affect the payment of your bill.
9. Don't give the debtor the option to say "No." Wishy-washy statements ("I don't suppose you can pay the whole bill now, can you?") just beg for a "No" answer.
10. Keep calm and polite. If the debtor becomes angry and shouts, never shout back. A fire dies down if you don't add fuel. Don't react in the way the debtor expects. He'll almost always cool off fast and apologize to you.

Collecting by phone is just a variation of the art of selling. First you sell yourself by your attitude, and then you sell your product, in this case, prompt payment of your doctor's bill. So to be a good telephone collector:

— Don't tear the patient down; build him up.
— Make him want to pay you. Persuade him by offering reassurance of your good opinion of him, providing a reason that is valid, and by restoring his self-respect.

Remember: **Everyone** pays **some** of his bills every month. Your job is to make sure that your bill becomes one of the important ones.

4

Investigating by telephone

"A wise man's precaution"

Far better than the eyeball test in determining the honesty and ability of your new patient to pay is the test made by ear, using the telephone. Does this mean buying a report from the local credit bureau? It may, if you practice in a small town where the bureau has a real handle on the paying habits of everyone. Otherwise, it doesn't.

Take a look at the credit report on page 36. Nothing on it could possibly help you learn how the subject's medical bills are paid. Therefore, if you were to depend solely on such a report, you would probably be misled. Reason: As we'll discuss later in the chapter, prompt payment of the type of bills listed in a credit report is not a true indicator of how this patient will pay **you.** So you must use the telephone to test the would-be patient. That involves verifying the information he gives you, determining as much as you can about his insurance coverage, and learning the experience of his previous doctor.

Of course, **you** don't have the time to do that yourself. Your assistant will have to do it for you. Be assured that it's not necessarily very time-consuming. Think of it this way: If your assistant has time to pursue patients who don't pay, and to keep rebilling them endlessly because she didn't take a few minutes to check them out at the beginning, she really can't afford **not** to have time.

Is all this a case of snooping into the affairs of the new patient? Not really. It's just a wise man's precaution, prior to investing possibly large amounts of valuable time treating a stranger.

This is an actual credit report with just the name changed to protect the privacy of the individual. Notice that although it goes back seven years or more, no medical credit information appears on it. While adequate for commercial credit granting, it is of little help to the medical business office.

CONFIDENTIAL *Factbilt* ® REPORT	FOR	Dr Roger Kildare	IN FILE SINCE: 1967

This information is furnished in response to an inquiry for the purpose of evaluating credit risks. It has been obtained from sources deemed reliable, accuracy of which this organization does not guarantee. The inquirer has agreed to indemnify the reporting bureau for any damage arising from misuse of this information, and this report is furnished in reliance upon that indemnity. It must be held in strict confidence, and must not be revealed to the subject reported on.

REPORT ON (SURNAME):	MR., MRS., MISS:	GIVEN NAME:	SOCIAL SECURITY NUMBER:	SPOUSE'S NAME
DOE	JOHN	J	101 22 6324	JANE

ADDRESS:	CITY:	STATE:	ZIP CODE:	SPOUSE'S SOCIAL SECURITY NO.:
1611 Dundee St	San Francisco	Ca	94117	---

COMPLETE TO HERE FOR TRADE REPORT AND SKIP TO CREDIT HISTORY

PRESENT EMPLOYER AND KIND OF BUSINESS:		POSITION HELD:	SINCE:	MONTHLY INCOME
CPA	Self employed		1967	$1500 est

COMPLETE TO HERE FOR SHORT REPORT AND SUMMARY REPORT AND SKIP TO CREDIT HISTORY

DATE OF BIRTH: 6-8-35	NUMBER OF DEPENDENTS INCLUDING SPOUSE → 3	☐ OWNS	☒ BUYING	☐ RENTS HOME

FORMER ADDRESS:	CITY:	STATE:	FROM: 35	TO: 67
14661 Glenfield,	Detroit,	Mich		

FORMER EMPLOYER AND KIND OF BUSINESS:		POSITION HELD:	MONTHLY INCOME	FROM: 60	TO: 67
Metts, Drake & Thompson	CPA	Accountant	$650		

SPOUSE'S EMPLOYER AND KIND OF BUSINESS:	DATE VERIFIED	POSITION HELD:	MONTHLY INCOME:	FROM:	TO:
None			$		

CREDIT HISTORY *(Complete this section for all reports)*

KIND OF BUSINESS	DATE REPORTED OR VERIFIED	DATE ACCOUNT OPENED	DATE OF LAST SALE	HIGHEST CREDIT	AMOUNT OWING	AMOUNT PAST DUE	TERMS OF SALE AND USUAL MANNER OF PAYMENT
DEPT	3-74	11-67	3-74	300	250	0	R-1
OIL/NATL	12-73	1-65		120		current	0-1
CLOTHING	9-73	11-67	9-73	400	330	202	0-5
CLOTHING	6-73	12-67	5-73	500	279	53	0-2
DEPT	1-73	12-69	12-72	125	0	0	0-1
CLOTHING	1-73	3-70	12-72	800	800	0	0-1
CLOTHING	1-73	2-72	12-72	93	83	0	0-1
SPORTING	9-72	12-69	11-69	220	0	0	0-0
BANK	9-72	11-67		2012	0	36/MO	1-1

PUBLIC RECORD AND/OR SUMMARY OF OTHER TRADE INFORMATION:

All previous trade as agreed. No court items of record. Nothing derogatory in file.

The remainder of this chapter is intended as instruction for your assistant. If you agree with the principle, you have only to ask that she follow the advice given. The result will be a certain decrease in the number of your delinquent accounts, and a corresponding increase in your income.

Advice to an assistant: How to detect deadbeats

As the doctor's assistant, you're vitally concerned with the no- and slow-pay patients in your ledger. That you're reading this chapter is proof that your doctor wants you to keep the number of such delinquents down.

Now for a moment of truth! Isn't it true that some of those delinquents with large balances wouldn't be in that ledger if you'd have caught them on the way in? In all probability, you didn't catch them because you didn't know what to look for. And that's what this chapter is all about.

By learning a few of the techniques you can become an investigator as good as those employed by your collection agency—and probably much more highly motivated. Why be so critical of the information given by new patients? What are the dangers you're supposed to be looking for? Here's a description of five common types that your new alertness can catch:

The Honest Nitwit. She's sure her insurance pays for everything, or that she still has coverage when, in fact, it's entirely used up. Her previous doctor or her employer's personnel office can easily clear this up for you.

The Proud Hero. She needs to lie about employment status. The self-proclaimed office manager, for instance, who is really a bookkeeper. The danger here is that you'll overestimate her income and extend more credit than you should.

The Window-Shopper. She tries out doctors the way she tries out restaurants. She has a chronic ailment but never stays with any doctor long enough for treatment. Getting no relief, she sees no reason to pay.

The Little White Liar. He registers truthfully when he fills out your form, except for one small thing—he claims to have insurance when he doesn't. Or says he's employed, when he isn't. Or that he lives at an address he moved from two months ago.

The Bunco Artist. His registration form is a work of art—complete fiction from first to last. Fortunately, he's not too common and he's easy to catch if you do any telephone checking at all.

Naturally, you want to catch these types on the way in, but how do you do it? Whom do you call? What should you ask?

For all new patients, the first call should be made to the personnel office of the employer reported.

You'll want to learn whether he really works there, is covered by group insurance, and what the coverage is. If there's a deductible, how much? And how much of it has been used up?

Quite often, the girl you first talk with won't know the answers. Remember, though, that you're about to extend credit on the basis of this information. You must have it. Your courage at this point is all that stands between your doctor and a potential financial loss. Tell her that you have to know and that you'll call back in 10 minutes. Tell her that it's important to the patient, who will need credit based on the information.

Sure you used up three or four minutes talking, and you'll use up three or four more when you call back. But you'd use up more than that if you billed an insurance company that wouldn't pay and then tried to collect from the patient.

What should you do if there's no insurance coverage, or if the balance after insurance will require the patient to seek credit? The very best information is how he paid his previous doctor. So, for patients who are going to need credit, make one more call. This is to your opposite number in the previous doctor's office, as shown on your patient's registration form. You'll need to know:

1. The patient's bill-paying record.
2. What insurance coverage he had.
3. His general attitude.
4. Whether he and his family missed or were habitually late for appointments.

The information you gain from this call is invaluable in assessing your new patient. In return, you'll offer the same service to the other assistant, if she ever needs it.

A point to remember: Under the Fair Credit Reporting Act, if you generally allow credit to your patients, you can't deny credit to one of them without telling him why. If your denial is based on a report from his previous doctor, you're required to tell him so. And any doctor who calls you for a similar report, and as a result denies credit to a patient, is required by law to tell that patient the source of his information—you.

Some authorities will advise you, for this reason, not to give out any information and so avoid angering an ex-patient. This is wrong thinking. It surely doesn't make sense—after you've been mistreated by a patient— to refuse a carefully phrased warning to a fellow physician out of fear. People need to become aware that if they don't play fair with one doctor they can expect their next doctor to find out about it and to act accordingly. More cooperation among doctors will tend to discourage abuses of credit privileges.

Tracing the skip

As you become more sure of yourself in these simple telephone investigations, you'll be tempted to find other ways to use your new-found skills. A very profitable area, if you can find a few extra minutes in the day, and one that will earn your doctor's admiration and approval, is skip tracing. A doctor is the exception rather than the rule if he's satisfied with the way a collection agency has been collecting those skips he's sent it. You're the first to learn that an account is a skip. It becomes apparent when your statement comes back, unopened. You're in the best position to find this skip, too, because the trail is still warm. What should you do first?

Examine the envelope and classify it. If marked "Address Unknown," "No Such Number," or, simply, "Unknown," it falls into a group that we call "mistakes." This could be an error **you** made in addressing the envelope, or in transcribing the information from the registration form to the ledger card. It may be an error, possibly deliberate, that the patient made when he filled out the form. It's easily corrected by checking back over your records. If the error is not yours, try calling one or two of the numbers he gave you. If you run into a dead end here you know you're in trouble, because if he deliberately tried to mislead you he's going to be extremely hard to collect from, even when you find him. On the other hand, if the patient just goofed, you'll be able to get his correct address from the people you call. Another method is to call telephone information and say: "I'd like the telephone number **and the address please** of etc." This may not always work.

A more common reason for your mail to come back is the case of a true skip. This mail is marked: "Moved, left no address," or words to that effect. Before you pass any final judgment on such a patient, remember that this could just possibly be an oversight on his part in failing to provide the post office with a change-of-address card. In that case, when you call up his closest relative you'll quickly learn his new address. If that's unsuccessful, try calling him at his work. He may have moved but still be working at the same job. If he's left, ask for his immediate supervisor. If the move was sudden he may have contacted his employer about a final paycheck. In any event, someone there may know where he went.

Here are some tips that may help you:

Let's suppose you draw a blank at the employer's. Call back and ask to speak to a friend. Say it's urgent. When you're connected, tell him that you're with the doctor's office, but not the reason for your call. If you can't draw him out, try getting in touch with neighbors. Don't refer to him in a derogatory way, or divulge what the call is about. It's poor business practice and quite dangerous to say anything that might be construed as damaging to another's reputation. Besides, it's poor psychology. People clam up if they suspect you're a bill collector. It's far better to appear to be a friend.

How can you find the names of these neighbors? Even in small communities you can subscribe to city directories that list the names of most residents by the streets on which they live. In many cities, the telephone company also makes a list of subscribers available, arranged according to address. In some larger cities, this information is available by telephone from the public library.

An advantage of living in a smaller community is that you can get on good terms with a girl in the phone company's business office, the electric company, or the water department. All these offices have information of this sort available, and are usually cooperative if they know that the information is to be used for a legitimate purpose.

If this initial investigation is unsuccessful and the size of the bill justifies more effort—and you have the time to spend on it—here are more sources of information to try:

— *Landlord of the property he lived in.* By phone, if an apartment house; by mail, if a single residence.
— *The Board of Education,* if he had children, to find out the school district he lived in and the closest elementary school. When you find this, call the office to learn a forwarding address. If no luck there, try the school nurse.
— *The police.* They may have a record of him. He may be on probation and have to report his new address to them.
— *The self-drive truck rental* nearest his former home. If he rented a truck, they'll have a record of his destination.
— If his last name is fairly unusual, check the phone book for others with the same name. Call and ask for him.
— If your registration form shows the name of his bank, call and ask if the account was transferred or is still open. This will tell you if he's still local and, possibly, where he went.

Tracing skips is really detective work. The more information you have, the better chance you have of cracking the case. So, even if you do nothing else, have a good, complete registration form. See that it's completely filled out by each new patient. Check it by calling a couple of the phone numbers given, and **save it.**

5

How to choose your collection agency

"Between the rock and the hard ground"

"Between the rock and the hard ground" is an old cliché, but it
succinctly describes the uncomfortable situation many doctors find
themselves in between the time an account becomes delinquent and the
time it's assigned to a collection agency. The question they ask
themselves is: How far do I really want to go to get those bills paid?

If you feel morally righteous about nonpayment, agencies exist that
will go to almost any lengths to collect for you, provided you're willing
to foot the bill. At the other extreme, it may be important to you that
your patients be handled very gently, even after they leave your hands.

Collection agencies also differ widely, especially in policy. You'll
feel happiest with the agency whose operating procedure most closely
meshes with your own. However, unless you have some genuine basis
for making a selection, you might just as well rely on the Yellow Pages.
If you've ever found yourself at loose ends in a strange city and used
that method to choose a restaurant, you'll agree there's just got to be a
better way.

There are some rules to help you get the most from any agency you
use. Let's assume you've mailed numerous statements, that you've
stuck multicolored stickers on them saying, "Please," "Have you
forgotten?" or "Unless this bill is paid within 10 days it goes to our
attorney!"—all to no avail. Should you turn the bill over to an agency?
Not yet. Make just one more attempt.

Sometimes my collectors come to me with an account that they've worked hard on. They've called, left messages, done this or that without result, and want to give up. I usually urge them to try once more—this time using a little imagination and a different approach. Perhaps calling the patient's wife on **her** job, leaving a message with a friend rather than a neighbor, or maybe just writing the debtor a personal letter. In many cases those extra efforts succeed in getting the debtor's attention at last, and the collection becomes routine.

So always make that one last attempt and tailor it to the individual case. Break the pattern. You're probably much too busy to get directly involved, but try suggesting this approach to your assistant. Try composing a special master letter for her to send to all debtors immediately before assignment to an agency. Or have her make one last phone contact before an account is assigned.

But make it an unshakeable rule that once this final action is taken, the account goes to an agency. That way you won't have to see it and decide all over again.

Question: Naturally, I'm reluctant to assign any of my accounts to a collection agency. Isn't there some way, something I could do first, to soften the blow? A sort of intermediate step, perhaps?

Answer: Yes. Use a precollection letter service.

This type of service involves sending the delinquent one or two letters warning him of a last chance before a collection agency takes control of the account. It's almost invariably a mildly worded notice designed not to antagonize the patient. But it carries a strong punch because it's prepared by the agency on its stationery, and mailed from its office. Here's how it works:

The agency agrees to mail these notices out, usually free of charge, with the understanding that if the patient still doesn't pay or make satisfactory arrangements the account will be assigned to the agency for collection. Getting a notice from a collection agency, no matter how mild, has a galvanizing effect on the delinquent patient. And obviously, if two letters from a collection agency don't shake him up, then nothing you might have done will work either. It's an excellent device for separating the "will-pays" from the "won't-pays."

On medical accounts, about 20 per cent of debtors either pay or arrange to pay when they get these notices.

Question: Why does an agency perform this service for nothing?

Answer: Because giving your patient one last chance to pay makes it easier for you to assign the account. And if he still doesn't pay, it means that the agency gets the account sooner than it otherwise might.

Question: But that still doesn't tell me **when** I should give my accounts to an agency.

Answer: To put it in a nutshell, assign your accounts as soon as it
becomes obvious that you can't collect them yourself. This point
may be reached after 90 days, four months, or even much longer.
Here are some criteria to help you decide:

a. You've gone through your usual billing series and have received no
   money and no communication from the patient.
b. The patient has told you he's not going to pay.
c. The patient has promised to pay many times, but never has.
d. The patient made partial payment once, but more than 60 days
   have gone by with no further payment or word.

A point to remember: The longer you wait, the less chance the
agency has of making the collection. This is because other bills enter
your patient's life and he tends to regard the most recent as the most
pressing. Also if he's moved, the trail gets cold, the clues disappear, and
he's just that much harder to find.

All that may help you decide **when** to assign, but how about **who**
and **what?** In England, they refer to the process of swift decision as
"grasping the nettle firmly." The nettle is a weed that bears leaves
covered with a fine hair. If you touch or brush against the leaves, the
hairs produce a painful sting. But if you grasp the leaves tightly, without
hesitation, you escape the sting. Determining to assign your nonpaying

Assignment schedule		
	Days after	Action
Regular accounts	30	Itemized statement
	30	First statement
	15	Second statement
	15	Telephone call
	10	Special letter
	20	Precollection agency letter
		ASSIGN TO COLLECTION
Skip accounts	30	Itemized statement
	5	First statement (returned)
	5	Telephone investigation
		ASSIGN TO COLLECTION
Payment plans	15	Payment is missed
	15	Telephone call or notice
	20	Precollection agency letter
		ASSIGN TO COLLECTION

patients to an outside party for collection requires you to be decisive. But there are exceptions.

You have patients who should never be assigned for collection, no matter how long they take to get around to your bill. The reasons may be of a practical kind, or there may be humane considerations. The patient may be your brother-in-law, or your wife's best friend. Perhaps the bill is owed by an elderly widow on a small, fixed pension, or a young couple you've known all their lives struggling to keep their heads above water. Such accounts should be carefully tagged so they don't accidentally get turned over to an agency without your knowledge.

Accounts with balances of less than $10 shouldn't be assigned. It's like using a cannon to shoot birds.

A precollection agency letter is prepared and mailed by the agency telling the patient to pay you directly or the account will be retained by the agency. If the patient pays or makes satisfactory arrangements, you may then withdraw the account from the agency, usually without payment of a fee.

Disputed accounts should be carefully analyzed before they're assigned. The agency will always assume that you, as its customer, are always right. This partisan attitude tends to infuriate an already disgruntled patient and may make a reconciliation difficult to achieve. On the other hand, if you've already clashed with your patient and feelings have been hurt, a good agency can often bring about satisfactory compromise. If that's the problem, be sure to let the agency know.

More difficult are cases in which the patient claims to have suffered damage from work you've done for him. In such a case, hasty assignment to an agency could push your patient right into the hands of an attorney. When that happens, you may not lose, but you can hardly ever win. The bill may be paid, but the cost to you in time and stress will far exceed any monetary gain.

Naturally, when you assign accounts, you expect to get results. On a national basis, though, only 28 per cent of all accounts assigned to agencies are presently being collected. This means that 72 per cent are being written off as uncollectible, and some of your accounts are almost certainly going to be among those failures. Those percentages are just averages, of course, and there are definite steps you can take to help your agency collect considerably more than that. Some agencies with which I'm familiar collect more than 50 per cent for some doctors. These doctors are usually more businesslike than most, and they tend to follow these basic rules:

1. Use a good, comprehensive, new-patient registration form.
2. Insist that the form be properly filled out by the patient.
3. Be decisive. Don't keep putting off assigning an account because

you think maybe a payment may come in next month.

4. Give the agency **all** the information you have when you assign the account. (This can double your chances of getting the account collected.)

Question: What should I look for when choosing a collection agency?
Answer: A high standard of ethics, a good record with other doctors, and an attitude toward debtors that's compatible with yours.

Most states have some sort of collection agency licensing bureau. In California, for example, the bureau sets rules for who may and may not operate an agency, and it requires every employe engaged in the collection or solicitation of accounts be registered with the bureau and not have a police record. In addition, the bureau requires that each agency or branch must be under the direct control of a manager possessed of certain stringent qualifications for operating an agency. And it holds this manager responsible for enforcing its regulations. It checks on his performance by making surprise audits from time to time, and follows up any complaint by either customer or debtor.

Although the basic processes of collection are similar, the manner in which they are carried out differs sharply among agencies. The style ranges from a bully and threat approach (accompanied by almost indiscriminate use of legal action), to the other extreme, which often consists of little more than sending out dunning notices.

In our experience, the medical profession particularly has several needs that must be satisfied during the collection process. They are:

— Protection of the doctor's public image as a humanitarian.
— Protection of the doctor's self-image through assurance that the agency will treat his delinquent patients decently.
— Protection from countersuit by an indignant patient.

Not all businesses have such needs, at least to the same degree. So there are agencies that take a very roughshod approach. A doctor would be foolish to employ one of them. It pays to check into the nature of the agency you're considering.

The agency salesman may be very persuasive, but he's not the man who will be handling or mishandling your patients. You need to find out what the manager and **collectors** at the agency are going to do and how they're going to do it. Will they:

— Put your accounts through a two-letter, precollection service prior to actual assignment?
— Give voluntary progress reports from time to time?
— Return accounts within a reasonable time if they can't collect them?
— Guarantee that no lawsuit will be filed against one of your patients without your express approval?

- Tell you just **how** collections are made, what procedures are used, and what is said to debtors?
- Send dunning notices that stream out of a computer impersonally, inaccurately, and too frequently, or do they tailor them to the specific situation?
- Handle any and all accounts, or do they discriminate in choice of customers? (If staff members seem concerned about their clients' ethics, it's a good bet they're also concerned about their own.)
- Provide an indication of their collection effectiveness, and a list of references? (Have your assistant check them out.)

You need an agency that collects effectively, but without repercussions—one that persuades rather than forces.

Look closely at the agency's rates. If you assign your accounts within a reasonable time and part of the agency's service is sending precollection letters, expect about 20 per cent of your accounts to pay or make satisfactory arrangements. After you assign the remaining 80 per cent, a good agency should give some allowance for size of account, freshness, or ease of collection. But an agency has to keep an average of about one-third to make a reasonable profit, and 50 per cent has become the national standard. So don't fall for the line of the hotshot who solicits your accounts for some remarkably low rate.

Systems have been developed through which—for a small fee paid in advance on each of your accounts—a series of computer notices is fired at delinquent patients. Besides paying in advance with no guarantee of results, the total cost will probably amount to almost as much as you would have paid a regular agency in the first place. And you'll end up having to assign most of the accounts anyway. So, in choosing an agency, look for these assets:

- It should have a good reputation among your colleagues.
- It should have a clean record with your state's licensing bureau.
- Its treatment of your patients should not reflect adversely on your own image, or that of your profession.
- Its fees should be in line with the effort needed to collect your accounts.
- It shouldn't be suit-happy, but should lean toward a more persuasive, saleslike approach.
- It should be agreeable and cooperative with you in the matters of progress reports and the routine cancellation of accounts.

The collection industry, like other businesses, is competitive. If you know what you want and won't settle for less, there's an agency that will provide it for you in order to get your business. You're the customer, and the choice is yours.

6

Collecting from attorneys

"Tell it to the judge"

If you practice in a small town you may wonder just what the problem is in collecting from attorneys. After all, attorneys are intelligent, well-educated businessmen—aren't they? How could collecting proper fees from them be a problem?

Usually it isn't—if you practice in a small town.

In larger towns and cities, however, where the professional community is not so closely knit, and where the average doctor seldom knows even the last names of all the attorneys, there are problems. And while the bad boys among them make up just a small minority, those who don't pay raise a doctor's hackles and blood pressure out of all proportion to the size of the bill. Perhaps a look at some of the more common complaints will make this easier to understand. They all involve attorneys who:

— order reports and don't pay for them,
— advise their clients not to pay you until **after** the trial,
— wait until the last minute to tell you about court appearances,
— don't hold a pretrial conference with you,
— demand last-minute examinations of clients without notice,
— won't pay for your courtroom testimony if they lose the case,
— ask you to testify in favor of their clients, regardless of facts.

That's not a long list, but to most doctors the real irritation lies in the lack of ethics they feel is being displayed by the offending attorneys. The attorneys themselves see it quite differently. Most small-town attorneys will deny that any such problem exists, and they're probably right—at least as far as their own town is concerned. That's because the doctors and lawyers may have grown up together, or belong to the same Rotary Club, or play golf with each other.

But the truth is that even in such a familiar situation, the problem can exist. It's all a question of your point of view.

Here's an excerpt from a letter written to me by a small-town attorney, an elected judge, highly respected by his peers. From personal dealings, I know him to be highly ethical.

> "The matter of an attorney's advising his client not to pay medical bills prior to the outcome of a trial, I do not regard as a medicolegal problem. I look at it as a service that attorneys provide for the doctor in that money owed by the patient to the doctor, which is strictly a credit service matter between the doctor and patient, comes to the attention of the attorney by virtue of the fact that litigation is involved.
>
> "Normally, the condition requiring treatment by the physician has been the result of an incident for which some third party is liable to the patient.
>
> "In these situations, it is common practice for the attorney to check with the doctor's office, and if there is any bill still owed by the patient at the time a recovery is made, the lawyer will then deduct that amount from the recovery and pay it directly to the doctor as a service and guarantee to the doctor that he gets paid.
>
> "While it is true that this may result in a delay awaiting outcome of the trial, the lawyer is, in effect, protecting the doctor to the best of his ability.
>
> "In many instances, the patient is unable to pay for his medical treatment except from the recovery, and in the event that the patient loses his case, the doctor may never receive payment, and this would not be the fault of the attorney, nor would the attorney have any responsibility."

This argument, of course, ignores the fact that many attorneys advise the client not to pay the doctor because they expect to sway the jury by asking the client on the stand: "Mr. Jones, isn't it true that you're still burdened by extremely large doctor's bills as a result of your accident?" Later, they put the doctor on the stand and ask: "Now, Dr. Smith, will you tell us exactly how much Mr. Jones still owes you for the treatment you gave him at the time of his accident? Just answer with the figure he still owes, please."

So all you get to say is the figure. You don't get to qualify it with the fact that he's never paid you a cent. That leaves the jury with the impression that the original bill was much larger and that the poor fellow has managed to whittle it down to the figure you stated. In his letter, my attorney also overlooks the fact that many patients **can** afford to pay the doctor at the time they are treated.

In larger cities, with thousands of attorneys and doctors, a more impersonal approach is possible. In many cases, there's no social contact between these professionals that might influence their actions. In fact, most of them commute from suburbs that lie many miles apart.

These attorneys are much more direct in stating their cases. One well-known attorney, who prefers to remain anonymous, put it this way:

> "You bet I tell my client not to pay the doctor until he can collect from the defendant! Hell, I'm representing him, not the doctor. If, in my professional judgment, it's to our advantage to go into that court with a stack of unpaid medical bills, then I'd be a pretty poor excuse for an attorney if I advised him otherwise.
>
> "Once the case is settled and the money received, if my client asks me to pay the doctor direct, then I will. Otherwise it's up to the patient himself. The settlement belongs to him, no one else, and what he does with it is solely up to him."

With most attorneys, whether they admit it or not, that approach makes sense. They vary in the degree of their paternalism, however, and many will either pay the doctor direct, or at least advise the client to do so when the settlement is received.

So, if one day one of your patients says he isn't paying because his attorney advises him not to, what will you say to him?

There's absolutely no legal reason why you shouldn't be paid. You rendered service to the patient, and unless there was some previous agreement, he owes you your fee. Some patients can be persuaded to pay prior to a legal settlement, or at least to make payments until the settlement comes in.

One argument is to suggest borrowing from a bank or finance company. In that way they'll get time to pay off the bill and you'll be paid. Some others will pay if you suggest, through your assistant, that unpaid accounts over a certain age are automatically assigned to a collection agency.

With surprising frequency these days, doctors assign quite large bills on which nothing has been paid. Along with the assignment will be the terse comment: "Attorney handling." The collector will call the doctor for some elaboration since, as he sees it, there's little point in sending the account for collection when an attorney has entered the picture.

The doctor's lament sounds something like this:

> "This patient says his attorney **told** him not to pay me until after the trial. That means I may have to wait years to get paid, and I **know** the patient has the money. Damn it, anyway—how would he like it if I told **my patient** not to pay **him?**"

Well, let's ask a good attorney for his reaction to that statement:

> "A lawyer's job is to prevent injustice, not perpetuate it. Were I the collection agency I'd 'take the case,' immediately call the lawyer, and (1) settle, or (2) refer it to **your** lawyer. If you 'run' when a lawyer's name is mentioned, then you do a disservice to **your** client and shouldn't be in the business! The lawyer who says, 'Mention my name and they won't dare sue,' is a phony!"

That's a direct quote from Melvin Belli, certainly one of the leading trial lawyers in the country today. His comment, of course, is directed to collection agencies that accept assignments of this sort from doctors. Unfortunately, while most agency operators recognize the truth of Mr. Belli's statement, economic considerations usually take precedence over ideals.

When the agency calls, the patient follows his attorney's instructions and tells the collector to take it up with that attorney. The attorney then tells the agency: "You can wait until the case is settled, or you can file suit and try to get a judgment against my client. Of course, I'll definitely file an answer."

While the agency can file suit relatively cheaply ($20 or $30, because it has an attorney on retainer), a trial is a different proposition. Should the case go to trial—95 per cent of an agency's normal suits don't—the agency is at a disadvantage because attorneys seldom include court appearances in their retainer agreements. The agency, therefore, has to come up with comparatively big money to get him into court.

Now, since almost all agencies operate on a contingency basis with the doctors—one-third to one-half the amount assigned—they get nothing unless they collect. What if they lose the case?

There's always that chance because, by the very nature of their business, agencies don't attract top-line trial attorneys. More often than not, the attorney they retain for their day-to-day business is either young and trying to get by while establishing a clientele, or a not overly successful older attorney who is happy to get the drudgery of collection agency work. If the agency loses, it's out the costs, which can easily total $200 or $300. And the agency earns no fee from the doctor.

On the other hand, by simply going along with the patient's attorney, the agency can arrange to have the money paid to it when the case is settled, and collect a fee from the doctor for doing really nothing. Even if they opt for trial, it may be calendared 12 to 18 months ahead and the patient's case may well be settled before then.

For those reasons, agencies rarely make these collections prior to the original settlement date. So it's not advisable to turn this type of account over to an agency at all.

If you can't persuade the patient to pay, try to protect your fee by asking the attorney to pay you directly from any money received in a settlement. But don't just call him and then sit back relying on his agreement. Like any other office, his is set up to handle certain things with some degree of automation. When the settlement comes in, a check will be drawn up (after deduction of his fee) and made out to the client. The attorney is not legally bound to remember you.

Get some form of written agreement from him. It's even better if you can get the patient's signature on a letter instructing his attorney to withhold the amount of your bill from any settlement received. Here's an example of a form you could use:

TO: Attorney José Doe

I, Beverly Beaujolais, hereby instruct you to withhold from any settlement, payment, or judgment you receive on my behalf, the amount of Three Hundred Dollars due and owing to Dr. Charles Brown for medical services rendered to me, and to forward this amount directly to him.

Beverly Beaujolais

I, Attorney José Doe, hereby agree to abide by my client's instructions and to withhold the above sum from any settlement, payment, or judgment I may receive on her behalf, and to forward this amount to Dr. Charles Brown.

Dated   Attorney José Doe

Make two extra copies, one for the patient, one for the attorney, and have the signed original to come back to you for your file. With a signed copy of this agreement in your possession, it's unlikely that you'll have any trouble getting payment directly from the attorney.

What about an attorney who owes you money himself for such services as reports, client examinations, or trial testimony? Here's a quotation from another attorney:

"I am somewhat distressed by your statement that 'some attorneys politely refuse to pay' for services requested of doctors. From personal experience I feel that if the service is requested by me, then I owe payment for it and must look to the client for repayment. I am doubtful that the problem is of the magnitude that you imply. I would think that all the doctor would have to do would be to threaten collection through the credit bureau and the attorney would pay forthwith."

That's a small-town attorney's viewpoint. It overlooks the emptiness of the threat to assign the account when made to a city attorney, and discounts the fact that the doctor will lose up to half his bill, as the agency's fee, if he does assign the account.

In trying to collect a doctor's court-appearance fee, I once got this nasty reply from a big-city attorney:

"No, I don't feel like paying Dr. Brown $250 for trial testimony that was absolutely worthless to me. As a matter of fact, we lost the case as a result of his testimony. That means my client got nothing and, being on a contingency fee basis, neither did I. All the time I spent preparing the case and in court was wasted, all because Dr. Brown gave testimony which was not favorable to my client. Then he expects me to dig up his fee. Well, nothing doing."

You won't usually get such a direct reply. Instead, your billings will be ignored, your calls won't be returned, and if you do manage to reach him, he'll blame his office help for not sending you a check and he'll promise to look into it. What can you do?

Once again, we don't recommend using an agency, for basically the same reason as before. The best course, in our experience, is to contact the attorney yourself by phone, even if you have to call him at home, and tell him that if your bill isn't paid within 24 hours you'll go to the judge who handled the case and to the bar association.

The attorney will no doubt become quite vituperative. But don't budge from your position, and don't compromise. Keep in mind that his ethics are at fault, not yours. And most of his fellow attorneys will back you up.

Another difficult area in dealing with some attorneys is their complete disregard for the value of your time. A common complaint among physicians is that they're not advised of pending court appearances until the last moment. This means a disruption of practice and a hurried reshuffling of patient appointments and even operating schedules.

Your answer should be a flat refusal to appear for the attorney. And you'll be quite justified. After all, why—at a moment's notice—should you have to put aside the needs of other patients just to accommodate the inconsiderate attorney of one who is involved in litigation? When you refuse, the attorney has the choice of having you subpoenaed and turning you into a potentially hostile witness, or getting the case rescheduled for a later date—one you'll have time to plan for.

Almost as objectionable is the attorney who calls the day before trial and insists that you examine his client immediately.

He does this with complete disregard for your convenience or that of your patients simply so he can state in court that you've seen his client recently and can testify to her condition. The fact is he forgot to set up an appointment. You're supposed to uncomplainingly shuffle other patients around in order to squeeze his client in this afternoon and then have your assistants rush, perhaps even work late, to get your notes transcribed in time for the court appearance the next day.

Once again, if your schedule is heavy, the only response to this lack of consideration is to refuse. The attorney will then have to get the trial recalendared. That may teach him a little consideration.

Pretrial conferences are another area of contention. But they are for your own good. The attorney has an opportunity to brief you about questions he plans to ask and to alert you to questions you'll face under cross-examination. Without such a briefing, your testimony may not sound as professional as you would like. Under expert cross-examination, without knowing what to expect, you may find yourself and your professional opinion in a bad light. This can only work to the detriment of patient and attorney. A conference also helps set the attorney straight on his own line of questioning and thus keeps him from wrongful assumptions that might lose the case.

The day will probably come when you'll run into the character who tries to persuade or bribe you to testify in favor of his client, without regard to the facts. Give that misbegotten excuse for an attorney the same short shrift you'd give anyone inviting you to rob a bank.

Our experience with attorneys has proven that the vast majority are ethical, easy to work with, and never a real problem to collect from. But bear in mind that the first concern of a good attorney is his client. This inevitably means an occasional clash of opposing interests. So let any attorney know early in the relationship that you're friendly, cooperative, but completely uncompromisable. Following are some suggestions to help you keep that irritating minority of attorneys in line:

— To avoid embarrassing confrontations, make your position on professional ethics perfectly clear early in the relationship.

— Once you've had a problem with an attorney, put him on a

cash-before-service basis. Insist that your fee accompany any request for a report.

— If you're forced to wait for payment after treating his client, require the patient to give you an assignment endorsed by the attorney.

— If an attorney fails to notify you of a court appearance until the last moment, refuse to appear. Require him either to subpoena you or to get the trial date recalendared.

— Insist on a pretrial conference prior to any court appearance.

— If an attorney refuses to pay your fee for a court appearance because he lost the case, let him know that you'll take it up with the presiding judge and the bar association.

7

Blue Shield

"The jolly blue giant"

Among health insurers, Blue Shield—with its 72 independent plans—towers high above its competitors. In total subscribers, together with its cousin, Blue Cross, it stands second only to the U.S. Social Security program.

True, it's broken down into local, independent plans. But considered in toto, Blue Shield covers more than 80 million subscribers in the United States and Canada. Those covered under Government health programs administered by Blue Shield account for millions more.

The individual member plans that make up Blue Shield design their own subscriber contracts on the local level. But they're all associated through a central organization—the National Association of Blue Shield Plans (NABSP)—governed by a 33-member board of directors, representing the individual plans. As members, the plans make regular reports to NABSP on their financial status and operations. In their behalf, NABSP meets with departments of the Federal Government, helps create the policies made on that level, and passes down instructions to the member plans.

NABSP imposes certain requirements on its members beyond financial statements and reports. These requirements may concern policy. One example is the Utilization Review Program—mandatory for all plans.

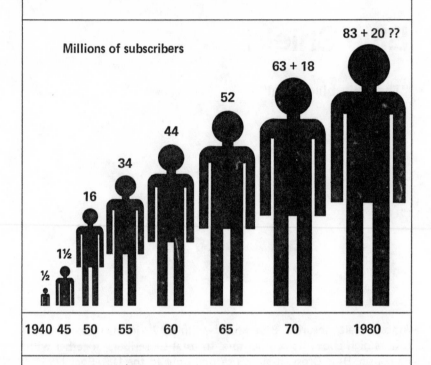

Growth rate of Blue Shield plans

Millions of subscribers

83 + 20 ??

63 + 18

52

44

34

16

1½

½

| 1940 | 45 | 50 | 55 | 60 | 65 | 70 | 1980 |

The chart covers the three decades ending with 1970, plus an educated guess for the increase expected by 1980. The plus figures shown for the 1970s and 1980s represent Blue Shield involvement in Government-sponsored health care. All other figures are membership in millions, as published by Blue Shield. The projected figures for Blue Shield's involvement with Government health care in the 1980s are certainly conservative. However, it's very likely that within the next 10 years at least half your patients will be covered, one way or another, through Blue Shield.

If size may be equated with success, the explosive growth of Blue Shield must be considered a great achievement, especially since it all happened within the past 30 years.

A proud claim made by Blue Shield representatives is that the cost of administering their program is held down to a skinny 11 per cent of subscriptions. Also, they're nonprofit-making.

For those reasons, it's in the financial interest of the taxpayer, as these Government programs proliferate, that Blue Shield be chosen to administer them.

Strangely enough, Blue Shield is not the child of the commercial business world. Its roots are in local medical associations, and doctors from those associations sit on the advisory board to this day. So, in a manner of speaking, it's your baby, doctor. The only trouble is that it has grown too big to hold in your own two hands. Plans and programs have increased to such an extent that the average physician grasps only the broadest outlines and finds himself at the mercy of remote boards which sometimes appear bent on perpetuating their own organization rather than solving problems of the individual M.D.

On the other hand, the plans offer almost any help you might ask for in the form of representatives, manuals, or newsletters. And many maintain professional-relations departments, available to answer your specific problem-questions.

Though these services still exist, some experts notice a shift in emphasis away from assistance and toward surveillance. They feel this shift is the result of economic pressure. Quite obviously, moving personnel from a department set up to help you file claims properly, to a department such as Utilization Audit Review, is bound to have a dampening effect on total volume of claim payments.

Considering this to be the reality of the situation, the wise course is to work within the organization. We suggest that you establish personal contact with someone in your local Blue Shield office.

You need a friendly business relationship with someone in middle-management in one of the departments that could help you, say, Medical Provider Services, or Professional Relations. It should be the kind of relationship in which you can lay your cards on the table and be confident that you'll get straight information in return. This will not only provide an interested party to check into a held-up claim, it will also put you in a position to learn about upcoming changes. Besides, you'll benefit from a more complete understanding of Blue Shield's own problems.

In any pragmatic evaluation of Blue Shield, it's important to keep two things in mind: Government participation in the medical field is here to stay; Blue Shield is destined to play a major part in administering that Government participation. You and Blue Shield will be working hand in hand for many years to come. It's only good business to learn as much as you can about your partner.

8
Government claims: Part I

"The Gordian knot"

Probably nothing else quite dulls the physician's eye or turns down his mouth so quickly as does a detailed discussion of the minutiae surrounding billing of Government claims. In this chapter we'll omit the wearisome details and hold the procedures for a later chapter intended just for your assistant. We will discuss the frustration underlying this outburst from an Ohio G.P.:

> "To tell the truth, all I **really** know about my Medicare claims is that a computer somewhere swallows them and months later—if I'm lucky—spits out a check for about half what my services are worth."

That sums up a sad situation, one that no doctor should tolerate for long. Reason? Because a clear understanding of this system of health care is vital to the financial good health of every physician now. And in the future, it will be an absolute necessity if he is to survive independently.

About 20 per cent of the claims being filed today are rejected and returned. This figure may vary, depending on the competence of your office. We know some offices that have reduced rejections to 2 per cent—a direct reflection of an unusually good grasp of the system.

What does a high rejection rate mean to you? At best, long delays in getting your money; at worst, lost income that you worked hard to get. It also means that you really can't be confident that your total accounts receivable figure is accurate.

The blame for this unbusinesslike situation can be shared fairly equally among the Government, your assistant, and yourself.

The case for the Government, as they tell it at Blue Shield, is the old three-headed hydra of fixed budget, expanding clientele, and rising medical costs. What recourse does Government have? Obviously, it can't spend money it doesn't have, so it's forced to tinker with the system in an effort to slow down the output. This shows up in frequent changes in requirements for eligibility and benefits paid. The changes filter down in the form of bulletins to the doctor that, unfortunately, his assistant doesn't have time to read. So they end up with Friday's garbage or—with the best of intentions—atop a stack of bulletins announcing all previous changes. Net result? Claims are filed incorrectly and are therefore rejected.

Rejections mean delayed payments, and delayed payments can be translated into borrowed time for the Government; time for demand to catch up with the supply of Government funds—bought at the expense of physicians.

That's Government's case, very fairly put, in my opinion, by a spokesman for Blue Shield. More than 60 per cent of Government claims are handled by Blue Shield. The remainder is parcelled out among a number of other large insurance companies. But the problem remains essentially the same, no matter who handles this Government business.

What part does your assistant unwittingly play in this conspiracy to keep you from getting paid? Actually, her situation is usually so difficult that it seems pointless to cast any blame. In too many cases, all she knows she received as a legacy from an ill-informed predecessor.

Since then, change has piled upon change so that, when the inevitable rejection comes in, she's understandably confused. Still, she grits her teeth and tries, depending on her own good common sense. Then, alas, when the claim is rejected anyway, she retypes it and tries again. Or, because she has a stack of ongoing claims to keep her busy, she puts the reject at the bottom of the pile to do "When I get to it." Either way, you're the loser.

The third partner in our conspiracy is you—the doctor. Let's look at what you may be doing that delays or even entirely disqualifies your payment.

If Blue Shield handles your Government claims, you talk to them and their computer through a set of 3,500 numbers called the Relative Value Studies, or R.V.S. Codes. Capricious use of these codes, I'm told, is the most serious cause for rejection of claims. So when using these numbers to describe treatment, degree of severity, and intensity of the patient's illness, you must be absolutely sure that they make sense when matched up with your diagnosis.

The codes are all that Blue Shield has to go by. When a clerk sees that these numbers correspond in only a peripheral way with your diagnosis, she's forced to conclude that you're mistaken, and changes the code. Naturally this situation becomes a problem to Blue Shield only when the amount you claim is higher than they think it should be. If a change is made, therefore, it invariably results in reduced payment to you.

Another cause for rejection is called "over-utilization" of the service. That means giving more medical care to an insured than Blue Shield thinks is appropriate. So that you won't feel that Blue Shield or any other carrier is being arbitrary when it reduces your fee on this basis, here's a statement by William C. White Jr., vice president for Government claims with Prudential Insurance Company, which shares a part of this Government business with Blue Shield:

> "It's almost impossible for the average doctor to avoid having at least some of his claims reduced. Remember, the carrier is responsible for determining the Government's liability under the insurance program prescribed by law. We are not necessarily judging a doctor's fee practices, or the way he practices medicine. The carrier, under this mandate, has to screen charges very carefully to decide if the treatment described was medically necessary. That's going to result in many reductions right there, because our medical staff may disagree with the attending physician— even after reviewing hospital records in some cases. Then, too, some doctors may consistently charge over the prevailing fee ceilings for their localities, even though they realize that their claims will be cut. If there's no Medicare assignment, they'll take their chances on collecting the remainder of their fees from the patients."

A rejection based on the charges Mr. White mentions is pretty sure to make you mad, but there's not much you can do about it. Decisions of that sort are made by what's called "the peer group," a board of physicians set up to review questionable cases.

Most doctors just don't realize how closely Blue Shield, or any other carrier handling Government claims, records their procedures and fees. To participate in the programs you must apply for a "provider" number from a carrier, which checks to make sure you have a medical degree and are properly qualified. Not so well known is the fact that the carrier also begins developing a profile of you and your practice.

In the credit-granting field, we say that a person creates his own credit record. A credit bureau doesn't rate people, but merely reports the history of their credit activity through the years. And this accumulation of facts speaks for itself.

Thus, it could be said that you build your own profile, procedure by procedure, and charge by charge, as you report them in your billings and claim forms.

In addition, Blue Shield develops at least two other profiles that it finds useful in judging your claims. One is the specialty profile, a constantly updated record of charges made by all physicians in a given specialty. The other is an area profile that includes all physicians practicing in a given region.

A physician can see his personal profile upon request. The specialty and area profiles are confidential. From the dollars and cents point of view, this secrecy on the part of the carriers is reasonable. Almost any doctor, if he learned that the majority of physicians practicing his specialty in his area were charging more, would be tempted to raise his fee level to match theirs.

How can a doctor find out what the local level in his specialty is? Can he find out by writing to his carrier? Mr. White of Prudential replies:

> "We wouldn't tell him. That's one of the few pieces of information that the Bureau of Health Insurance won't let us divulge to anyone. Prevailing charge levels are based on customary charges, and those charges do vary among physicians. Then, too, the fees for Medicare cases are not supposed to be higher than those for non-Medicare patients. Each doctor establishes his fees according to his own situation, and he should have freedom to do just that.
>
> "On the other hand, you can't ignore the very human stimulus there'd be to raise fees to the prevailing levels if those levels were published or openly broadcast. And if all the doctors moved to those levels, then we'd have, in effect, a national Medicare fee schedule. The long-range implications of that, I believe, would be detrimental to both doctors and patients."

These profiles are why one doctor may tell you he's getting paid "100 per cent across the board" for Medicare cases, while another complains that he's getting only 65 per cent of what he bills.

The carriers will never voluntarily increase your Medicare fees. If you're receiving very close to the amount you bill, don't feel too smug about it. That friend of yours who wails that he's getting only 65 per cent may still be getting more than you—if his profile was established on a higher fee schedule than yours.

So much for fees. There's another problem right in your office that may insidiously lead you to believe that you're in better shape financially than you really are. That can be dangerous. Here's the problem: Unless you're an exception, you don't have an accurate idea of how much is outstanding on your books, and you have no way to find out. Reason? With Government billing, you can't accurately predetermine how much you'll actually receive. For example:

On some of your ledger cards, a balance will show up after Blue Shield's payment, reflecting a reduction made in your charge. On others, no payment will have been received because the claim was rejected, but no record of this rejection shows on the card. Still others will show an unpaid, pending balance from Blue Shield, the amount of which you can only guess at.

Unless you're on the ball and keep separate books for your Government billing—having your assistant go through them regularly charging off uncollectible balances and keeping close track of accounts on which final rejections have come in—you'll never know your true receivable figure.

Mishandled receivables are a real headache, so have your assistant set up the system recommended in the special chapter of instruction beginning on page 68 that we've included for her. It's designed to give you a true picture of receivables due you from Government billing.

To sum up the problems with Government claims:

1. They won't stand still long enough for you to draw a bead on them.
2. They tend to distort your accounts receivable.
3. The carriers cut down and reject your charges in an arbitrary way.

The answer to Problem 1 is in the next chapter. Problems 2 and 3 can be greatly alleviated by allowing your assistant to follow the directions given in her special chapter.

9

Government claims: Part II

"Questioning your paycheck"

The real solution to getting your fees paid is understanding just how the carriers calculate the amount they pay you, and what you can do if you don't like it.

The standard method of determining payments used by all insurance carriers that handle Government claims is called the median technique. At one time, some carriers used as a base the charge you made most frequently for a particular treatment. Other carriers depended on averages. Today, all use the median—the numerical midpoint (not the mean) of all your charges for a specific service during a given time period.

How a fee profile is shaped

Dr. A's charges for an office visit range from $7 to $10. The insurance company's computer lists, in ascending order, all the office visit charges that appear on his claims. Then it locates the median, or midpoint, of those charges, thus:

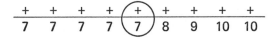

For Medicare purposes, the median figure of $7 becomes the customary charge in Dr. A's fee profile. If the median should fall between the two different charges—$7 and $8—the customary fee would be the higher figure. This method is used to compute all of Dr. A's customary charges, and the profile is stored in the carrier's computer for reference. Unless this figure is higher than that charged by others in his specialty in the same locality, it's used in determining payment of his claims.

That doesn't mean you actually get the median fee. Your median is compared with customary charges for your specialty in your designated locality, and adjusted accordingly. A locality is defined in many ways, but must include an economic cross section of the population. It's usually an economic or political subdivision of a state.

The carriers determine the localities. For example: They may decide that a state should have five localities for G.P.s, but use the entire state for a particular specialty because there just aren't enough of those specialists to justify a smaller area.

Doesn't this work to the benefit of the carriers and against the doctors? In a way, yes. But without it, the prevailing fee standard would be meaningless, because of the wide discrepancy in the fees charged in different localities.

How prevailing fees are determined

In 1971 the Bureau of Health Insurance arbitrarily froze Medicare physicians' fees at the 75th percentile of charges submitted during 1970. This means that a doctor can collect 80 per cent of his customary Medicare fee only if that customary fee doesn't exceed the highest fee being charged for the same service among three-fourths of the doctors in the same locality and field of practice.

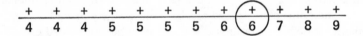

Any G.P. whose profile for an office visit doesn't exceed $6 can collect 80 per cent of his customary charge from Medicare, up to a maximum of $4.80 (80 per cent of $6). However, Dr. A in the previous example, assuming he's a G.P., collects only 69 per cent of his customary fee because it's higher than the top charge among three-fourths of his colleagues. In short, he gets 69 per cent of $7, or $4.83.

Obviously, what you charge has an effect on your profile, and all doctors are not paid the same. What can you do to raise **your** median? Raising all your fees across the board will not, in itself, do it. Not, that is, unless you can convince your carrier that such an across-the-board raise is essential to your practice.

To do that you'd need as much evidence as possible that your existing profile is too low. You must show that you're working at a high level of productivity, but still suffering financially. You have to prove that your income has dropped, or that you can't keep up with your overhead.

You could document this with such things as rent increases, building improvements, equipment purchases, higher salaries, or the necessity for hiring additional assistants—all the kinds of expenses that drive up practice costs. Even presenting all this material won't guarantee increases, but it will help your chances more than anything else. Of course, your case would be looked upon much more favorably if you hadn't increased your fees for a significant period—at least a couple of years.

Make your request to the carrier's regional office, the one through which you've been sending your claims. In your letter, state that you plan to raise the fees you've listed. These could be part or all of your schedule. Specify the date on which the fees will be raised and request that your fee schedule be raised to reflect them. Include your documented reasons.

Your request will be reviewed by a member of the carrier's staff—usually someone familiar with your profile and claims history. If he has any questions, he'll call or write before making his recommendations to higher levels within the carrier's organization.

Should your request be turned down, you can ask for a meeting with someone on the carrier's staff and get another chance to argue your case. Sometimes they won't grant your total request; they'll compromise on a raise of some sort.

If your request is approved, you must charge the new fees for three months before you get any additional money from the carrier. And if you've already bumped up against the prevailing fee ceiling for a given service within your locality, the change won't bring you higher payments from your carrier.

Are you eligible for a fee rise?

	YES	NO
No raise for over two years.	☐	☐
Productivity the same or increased.	☐	☐
Expenses demonstrably increased.	☐	☐
You're hurting financially.	☐	☐
You're below the prevailing fee ceiling.	☐	☐

Total

The higher the number of "Yes" checks, the better your chances. However, even a "No" on the last two won't necessarily disqualify you.

Once established, your profile is fairly permanent. But it can be changed by circumstances and situations. For example: If you moved your office from one Medicare locality to another, your profile would be recalculated from scratch according to the new locality's schedule of prevailing fees.

About the only way to find out the prevailing charge levels in a new area is to check with established doctors there in your own field of practice. The carrier will refuse to give this information, claiming that the Bureau of Health Insurance forbids it.

One of a doctor's biggest frustrations results from reduction of a claim. To improve your chances of getting the full allowance, make sure that your claim reflects the full extent of the service. It definitely pays.

Make sure your claim reflects the full extent of the service

Part II — (Physician or supplier to fill in 7-14)				
(7) a Date	b Place	c Fully describe surg. or medical treatment	d Nature	e Charges
3-6-71	I.H.	Reduction *INCORRECT*	Fx Femur	$600

3-6-71	I.H.	Open reduction with pinning *CORRECT*	Fx Femur	$600

The first form is incorrectly filled out. The prevailing fee for a reduction in that area is $300. Carrier will reduce fee to that figure. The correct description in this case would have been: "Open reduction with pinning." In that case, the higher figure would have been allowed. The inadequate description cost the doctor half of his rightful fee.

If one of your claims should be reduced, and you consider the reduction unfair, you can always ask the carrier to review its decision. If that doesn't work, you can ask for a hearing. The hearing must relate to a specific claim; it can't be an over-all review of your fee profile or claim reductions.

The carrier will designate someone to conduct the hearing who was not involved in the original processing of the claim. The hearing is your right, but it's unlikely to do you any good. If the carrier made an error, chances are it would have been caught when you first complained. The hearing officer's decision is final; no appeal is permitted.

How to stay on top of your Government claims

1. Find out what your carrier uses as "customary fee" for your most frequent charges.
2. At every opportunity, find out from your colleagues in the same specialty what they usually charge for the same procedures. Rough out your own "area profile."
3. If your fee schedule is below that of your colleagues, take the steps outlined to request an across-the-board increase.
4. Be very explicit in describing your treatment on a claim form. Don't take the chance of being paid for a less extensive treatment.
5. Establish a contact on the staff of the carrier. His advice can save you mountains of red tape and many pointless hearings.

10

Government claims: Part III

"Advice to an assistant"

When it comes to Medicare, Medicaid, or any other Government-sponsored program, red tape and constant change are the order of the day. Your skill and imagination in handling these claims will determine how much your doctor gets paid on them and, indeed, whether he gets paid at all.

You may already run a tight ship, be up to date on all current changes, and know to the penny how much you'll be paid on each claim, and seldom get a rejection. If so, you're worth your weight in gold.

The vast majority of assistants, however, have trouble with Government claims. And no wonder.

Usually, when an assistant starts her job, there are so many other things to grasp all at once that she never has time to sit down and study all the rules and requirements for preparing these claims. As a result, she's not really sure of herself, and her doctor never gets as high a return for his work as he should.

If that brief description fits you, we can offer some help. The instructions that follow are general; it's up to you to tailor them to the needs of your office. Once you get things organized properly, you'll manage the job in less time and the guilty feeling of being behind in your work will be lifted.

Before we delve into the details of what you **should** do, let's look at some of the more common troubles. See if you recognize any:

Charges not posted to a claim form. A patient is seen and charges are made—but they're never posted on a claim form. As a result, the carrier doesn't get billed. So the doctor doesn't get paid.

Wrong number used. The numbers from the patient's I.D. card aren't copied correctly. Result: The claim is rejected. If you can't reach the patient, the doctor doesn't get paid.

Illegible handwriting. Most claims are still filled out by hand and the writing often defies deciphering. The claim may be rejected or misread. Either way, your doctor loses money.

Typographical errors. Strikeovers, misspellings, transpositions—all can make forms invalid, cause rejections, cost you and the carrier time and your doctor money.

Bulletins and newsletters not read. Required changes are missed and so claims are improperly filled out. Much time is wasted and money lost in trying to correct this common error.

Poor record-keeping. Charges, payments, write-offs aren't properly posted to patient cards. Result: You don't know what's to be paid, what has been paid, what never will be paid.

Patients misinformed. Assistant unable to provide correct information to patients. Result: difficulty in collecting balances after insurance.

Accounts receivable questionable. Carrier's partial payments and rejections not noted, or uncollectible balances still carried forward. All combine to distort the receivables. Result: trouble for the doctor if he puts any faith in your figures.

Admittedly, that list represents the worst offenses, and I'm sure you won't find them all in your office. But you may recognize one or two. If so, face the fact. With a little better organizing you can eliminate the loopholes. We offer the following procedures:

Setting up a claim

Make up your claim form on the first day that the patient comes in each month. This is a must. If your carrier requires you to use a label, stick it on the form. Type in the name, address, date of birth, cause of condition, and similar items. Enter the treatment given, in detail. Put in the date, procedure numbers, description, place of treatment, and the charge. Leave the form in the patient's folder. Should the patient come in again during the month, add the charges that same day.

Completing the claim

Keep all claim forms of patients on Government insurance separate from non-Government forms. On a designated day at the end of each month, pull out all the forms, check to be sure they're complete, and have the doctor sign them. File all office copies alphabetically in a separate file. Don't put them back in the patients' charts. Label them. For example:

"Government Claims, Pending May, 1974"

In this way you're creating a built-in aging system for follow-up in case of nonpayment. As payments come in, pull the copy of the claim form, staple the information part of the check to it, and place in a file marked:

"Government Claims, Paid"

Adjusting your accounts receivable

In posting to your books, use four columns for entries—debit, credit, adjustments, balance. Then, when a Government claim falls short—and you're not permitted to collect the difference from the patient—use the adjustments column to write it off. Don't keep a running balance, month-to-month; balance out each month.

By handling your Government claims in those ways, you'll never be carrying forward an inflated total that includes balances that will never be paid. Your doctor will then be able to judge his receivables much more precisely.

11

Doctors Organized for Credit

"What's up, DOC?"

Individually, doctors are small-business men—at least in the eyes of the credit and collection industry. And there's not much one doctor can do to change that.

Consider his relationship with a collection agency: The average doctor may assign $300 or $400 in accounts a month, at the very most. The agency can forget about 20 per cent of this figure as collected by free, precollection letters, and about the 50 per cent of the remainder that's statistically uncollectible. (Nationally, only 28 per cent of all accounts assigned to agencies are collected.) At a collection commission of 50 per cent, that leaves a return to the agency of no more than $80. That's not enough to make an agency change its traditional policy to please any one doctor.

So, even if you try to get some of the programs mentioned in this book installed by your agency, you'll probably fail. You just don't have the leverage. Groups or clinics have more, of course, but even they would have a hard time reversing a large agency's cement-hard standard procedure.

What does that leave? Well, if you feel, as do many doctors, that you've been shortchanged by the credit and collection people, look into a new concept called "Doctors Organized for Credit," otherwise known as DOC.

This concept is based on leverage. All doctors in a given area (a county, say) hire a medical management consultant to represent them in dealing with collection agencies. They give him a list of requirements;

he analyzes the agencies in the area and chooses the best.

He then offers DOC's entire collection business—it should amount to more than 90 per cent of the medical collections in the area—if the agency will accommodate to the doctors' needs. In some cases, DOC members may decide to use two agencies. That provides a basis for comparison of results and serves to keep both agencies hopping.

It works because the heart of the collection agency world is competition. All agencies field salesmen and wage a continuing struggle to hang on to clients and to wrest new ones from other agencies. The struggle is necessary because of the very narrow margin of profit, and the tendency, in this consumer-oriented age, of legislators to work to the advantage of debtors. So, when something like DOC comes along with an opportunity to tie up all the medical business in a county while reducing or eliminating need for a sales force, it's enough to shake an agency right down to its tradition-bound foundation.

How good is a medical business, qualitatively, from the agency's point of view? Usually, very good, indeed. The lack of collection experience in the doctor's office usually makes it comparatively easy business to collect.

How much does an agency keep?	Assigned monthly	Collected through letter service*	Statistically uncollectible**	Your 50% share***	Gross return to agency
Small practice — $	100 $	20 $	40 $	20 $	20
	200	40	80	40	40
Large practice —	300	60	120	60	60
Group —	500	100	200	100	100
	1,000	200	400	200	200
Small clinic —	2,000	400	800	400	400
Large clinic —	5,000	1,000	2,000	1,000	1,000
Hospital —	20,000	4,000	8,000	4,000	4,000

*A good, two-letter service, sent out on the agency's stationery, should collect about 20 per cent of the accounts you list.

**The national collection average for accounts of all kinds was 28 per cent in 1971. Doctors' accounts are more collectible than the average.

***This comparison assumes that your collection fee is 50 per cent. If less, you may be paying in some other way, or getting less than full service on your accounts.

Consultant's services and fee

The consultant's fee varies according to the number of doctors in your association and the special services required. As a rule of thumb, the fee shouldn't exceed the savings that result from the lowered commission rate and the free, precollection letter service. His services may include:

Initially: 1. A written analysis of area agencies with recommendations for the selection of one or two.

2. A detailed, written presentation of your requirements to the chosen agencies.

3. Establishment of a Medical Information Center.

Monthly: 1. A written analysis of the collection effectiveness of the chosen agencies, individually broken down for each DOC member.

2. Supervision of the Medical Information Center.

3. Liaison between DOC and the agencies.

Special: 1. Individual and separately billed consulting for doctors whose return from the agencies is lower than the association average.

2. Research into other possibilities for DOC, such as cooperative medical equipment supply, or centralized Government claims billing.

The proof is that more agencies specialize exclusively in medical business than in any other single type of collection. So DOC's leverage in any community with more than one agency is very strong. It puts the doctor in the healthy position of being able to dictate the agency's commission rate. He no longer has to settle for a flat 50 per cent. (But don't expect Class A service for under 40 per cent because the agency's profit margin comes into play at that point.) And DOC also allows you to demand some valuable prerequisites.

If you've not been enjoying a free precollection service, make that one of your requirements. If you'd like to receive regular written progress reports, that also can be made part of the package. Perhaps you'd like some say about the wording of the notices the agency sends out, or some control over the legal action it takes. As a matter of policy, some agencies don't make out bankruptcy claims for you on patients assigned to them. But that's another requirement you can impose.

On those accident cases that you finally, reluctantly, assign because the patient's attorney says, "No payment until the case comes to trial," you can prearrange to withdraw if the agency fails to show prompt results. After all, you can sit on the file until after the trial just as well as the collection agency. And if you choose, you can build in the right to withdraw accidentally assigned accounts, and allow the agency only a nominal fee for its paperwork.

Whatever else may have bothered you in your relationship with collectors in the past can be rectified in the contract you write. That's something you couldn't do without the power and leverage of DOC. And the best part is that the whole process is painless. The consultant does all the work. All negotiating with the agencies is done through him. No one bothers **you**.

Another service that would make doctors happier is some sort of
medical credit-checking service. Many doctors have been frustrated
through the years because there's really no way to check out a new
patient's medical bill-paying habits. Credit bureaus may be of some help,
but the retail credit records they compile don't really reflect a patient's
paying record as it applies to his doctor.

Needed is a special service for the medical field. Fortunately, this
service can be provided in the form of a Medical Information Center,
through your association with DOC. It can be arranged through the
cooperation of your local credit bureau, through a collection agency,
or an office set up by a group of doctors. It requires neither large staff,
previous training, nor large initial investment. It works best, and is
least expensive, if set up as a small attachment to an existing

Requirements for a Medical Information Center

Space   Room for a desk and filing cabinet.

Equipment A used desk, chair, filing cabinet, desk-top file box, and a two-line telephone with hold button.

Personnel One clerk. (Can be employed doing other work at the same time she's on phone-answering duty.)

Supervision Your DOC consultant can be asked to make this part of his service.

Usage   One M.I.C. sponsored by 4 hospitals, 3 clinics, and 44 independent physicians and dentists averaged 55 calls a day. Each call took about 2 minutes.

Cost   In this M.I.C., the clerk was already on a payroll, so no fringe benefits were required. Her time was charged to the association at the rate of two hours a day. The office space and equipment were donated. The telephone cost about $20 a month. Total cost in this case was held to approximately $160 a month. This is probably a minimum. A figure of $300 to $400 would be more representative.

establishment. It could easily be a service rendered in a clinic or hospital.

It's easiest to organize in smaller communities; most difficult in large cities where the population is often transient and the large community of doctors presents problems in organization. To be effective, the center really needs at least 90 per cent participation. But if your community is of manageable size, and if the local medical professionals are a reasonably harmonious group and you can get them organized for their mutual benefit in an association such as DOC, setting up a Medical Information Center is really quite easy. All it requires is a 3" x 5" card file, filing cabinet, telephone, and an operator.

The alphabetically filed card system is simple enough, and the information on the cards is coded and confidential. Only your officers have a key to the code; the operator does not. The code consists of three letters and three figures, giving the patient's insurance information, paying record, and attitude. A number on the right-hand side of the card is the reporting doctor's identification number. A doctor inquiring about the patient could call the other doctor for more details. Or his assistant might call to get an insurance company name, or to find out if a balance remained unpaid.

The trick, of course, is getting such a service started. Most doctors want it when it's suggested to them, but seldom have the time to organize it. That's where your consultant comes in.

It's important to get the service started properly, making sure that uniform procedures are used for the correct input of information. Correct input is vital. In the press of day-to-day practice, some doctors tend to forget. If safeguards and controls aren't geared to feed information in smoothly, it's easy to become lax. An impartial third party, such as a consultant, can usually solve that problem without creating any hard feelings.

Once the service is set up, your assistant merely calls and gives the name and address of the patient she's checking on. The operator simply reads her the coded numbers. Your assistant then records these numbers on the patient's chart, and presto, you have a thumbnail sketch of what to expect. You also get the name of his previous doctor, information he may not have revealed to you. Knowing makes it possible for you to confer with the other doctor on subjects other than the patient's paying habits. The monthly membership assessment is your only cost for this.

To check on payment of assessments, the operator at the center maintains a card file of member doctors. When a doctor's assistant calls in after the first of the month, the operator checks the card file, and if the assessment hasn't been paid, she's not permitted to give out any further information until it is.

Monthly assessments are banked by the operator in a trust account, and a selected doctor (with a good bookkeeper) has power of attorney to write checks against the account to pay bills for the center. Initially, at least, all these charges would be small. The operator, for example, usually does other work for her employer during the hours she works the center—perhaps only four hours a day. Her cost to the members, then, would be minimal. Any surplus in the trust account can either be refunded to members at the end of the year, or accumulated to cover later expenses as the service grows.

Beyond collection control and credit information, there are numerous other possible uses for DOC. One is a central cooperative medical supply house, owned by the members. By combining buying power and eliminating middlemen, considerable savings can be realized.

Another might be a central office for Government claims billing. Much of the problem doctors are having with these claims could be eliminated if a team of experts handled them. The advantages of prompt

How a Medical Information Center works

Prepare and send in 100 3" x 5" cards with information on patients taken from your recent closed files. Then, once a week, have your assistant prepare cards on patients as you conclude their treatment. At first, she'll also include longtime patients as she handles their charts.

Pay your monthly, prorated assessment for the financial support of the center. Your share should certainly fall below $10 a month—a good investment compared with using regular retail credit bureau reports that cost from $.65 to $1.50 a call and which provide far less, if any, medical credit information.

The cards and monthly assessment are the sum total of your contribution to the center. In return, you have the right to call the center as many times as you wish, and request coded information on any person.

payment and reduction of rejected claims would more than make up for your share of the cost as a member of DOC.

Perhaps you're thinking that you don't want to get involved in trying to set these things up and worrying about them as they get started; that you have neither time nor inclination for this kind of business management. You're not the only doctor who feels that way, but there are always others who enjoy the challenge of this kind of enterprise. So don't let this become a deterrent. Usually, all you have to do is lend your support just by being a member, leaving the work to others more interested in it.

Doctors have traditionally shied clear of tight organization, preferring to hang on to their treasured independence. Nevertheless, there are some areas in which, without giving up a speck of independence, a doctor can benefit his practice and relieve his mind of nonmedical problems. The concept of DOC is certainly one of them.

12

Small claims

"Squeezing blood from a turnip"

Sooner rather than later, you're almost certain to become personally involved with a patient who won't pay, and who may even laugh in your face about it.

Perhaps you've tried to reason with him, and he's said, "Well, that's too bad, Doc. You're going to have to wait until I get good and ready to pay, which just may be never—and there's nothing you can do about it!" Sometimes, even after assigning the account, the agency will also be unsuccessful in collecting and tell you that the amount is too small to justify a suit. What's to be done?

You could try another agency, but chances are that it would also come to the same conclusion. You could get your attorney to handle it, but he won't do it for nothing. You'd also have to advance the court costs. And if the account is disputed, the debtor will probably get an attorney of his own and file an answer. That means a trial.

A trial can be expensive and time-consuming. Sure, if you win, the judge will usually award you the costs you've expended—which simply means he'll say that the debtor must reimburse you for them. But **you'll** have to collect from him, and that can take time. Meanwhile, those costs have come out of your own bank account.

The solution, of course, is to use small claims court, where costs are minimal and the judgments are as valid as those of higher courts. Neither collection agencies nor attorneys are allowed to take a case into a small claims court. Just you (or preferably your assistant) and the debtor appear before the judge. You state your case, and present your evidence. The defendant presents his side, and the judge makes a ruling. That's all.

In perhaps 9 cases out of 10, the defendant "chickens out" and doesn't appear. When that happens, you win by default. You still don't have any money, but you do have a legal judgment against the debtor and the right to "levy" against any assets he may have, such as his paycheck. That puts you in precisely the same position had your attorney handled it for you through a higher court—except financially. You've saved about $40 in out-of-pocket costs.

To file in small claims you have to pay a very small filing fee, in some courts as little as $1. You also have to pay a service fee to have the sheriff or constable serve the debtor with a summons. This amount varies from one part of the country to another, and according to the mileage the sheriff has to travel. It averages something over $3; seldom more than $10. Ask your attorney what it would have cost you to have him handle it through a higher court.

What happens when the debtor shows up? Occasionally, he'll come out of ignorance. He doesn't dispute the charge and has no defense except the lack of money to pay you. He's there only under the mistaken belief that he has to show up. He doesn't know that he could have let it go by default. He'll present no problem to you.

Sometimes, however, especially if he is a "big-mouth," the debtor will appear and try to talk his way out of paying. He may say that he has already paid, or that you overcharged him, or that he didn't agree to the service you gave to one of his dependents. But, you've had the opportunity to talk first. So simply state that the defendant refuses to pay you. Hand over your supporting documents—a copy of your ledger card, the original patient registration form he signed, dishonored check if any, and any letter he may have written concerning the account.

Unless he can come up with evidence that conflicts with yours, you'll win. To prove that he has already paid, he must have a canceled check or a receipt. He can't deny having had your services because the registration form he signed proves that he was in your office. As a general rule, judges will accept your office records at face value. That's why it's good business practice to keep legible, dated records of each effort— notices and phone calls—you've made to collect. Should the debtor claim that you overcharged him, the judge may question your assistant. So it's wise to inform your assistant, before she goes to court, about the treatment you gave.

No matter what the defendant says, don't speak to him directly. Address all your answers to the judge. Speak in a calm, controlled voice, and stick to the facts. Don't become annoyed, and don't waste the court's time with your opinions. Let the defendant be the one to make those mistakes.

In a small claims case, there is no appeal from the judge's decision. This cuts both ways, but the odds are in your favor. You have written evidence. You're calm and unruffled. You can answer the judge's questions clearly and logically. Right is on your side.

The mechanism of the law is constantly evolving, and small claims law is more progressive in some states than in others. In Oregon, for example, the limits have been raised to $500. The debtor may demand a jury trial and thus push the case into a higher court which will require both sides to be represented by attorneys. That's just as expensive for him as for you. So if he knows he owes you the bill, he's not likely to make this request. Debtors who insist on a jury trial are seldom the same people who receive a small claims summons because of an unpaid doctor's bill. Much more often it's something more contestable, such as a disputed claim for damage to a rented apartment.

Why you shouldn't appear in small claims court

If you get yourself involved in filling out forms, running down to the courthouse, and attending the hearings as they come up, you'll be wasting more time than the claims are worth. This is just as true of insurance claims, if you allow yourself to get caught up in the clerical work. So don't do it. One of your assistants is fully capable of handling the entire project for you, and attending all the hearings in your behalf. She'll find it quite simple after she's done it once.

Even if you lost every case in which the defendant actually appeared, you'd still win in the 9 out of 10 times he doesn't show up.

The judgment you get isn't worth a nickel unless you do something about it. The small claims office, usually right outside the courtroom, will gladly show you how to make out an execution of your new judgment.

If you choose to execute against your debtor's checking account, you'll make out an Execution Against Property form, showing the name and address of the bank he uses. And if you can get his checking account number, use it. It pays to be very sure that his name is filled in completely and correctly. One letter wrong, and the bank may say that it has no record of such a person. Specify the date of the judgment and the day it's to be served. It's effective on that day, and you don't want it the day **before** payday.

What if he's out of work and doesn't have a checking account? Well, judgment is good for a long time—10 years in most states—so you can afford to wait.

Does using small claims mean that you're stooping to methods properly reserved for tenement landlords and small-loan sharks? Definitely not. The small claims court system is the people's court; probably the most democratic of our legal institutions, and one of the fairest.

Though the matters at issue are small and comparatively inconsequential, it's here that one sees the purest form of our system of justice at work. The judge actually judges. He doesn't seem to be so bound by tradition and conformity as he is in the higher courts. There's room for a little humor, and with humor comes humanity.

Attorneys, generally, are not enthusiastic about small claims court because every time a potential client uses one, a possible fee flies out the window. You might feel the same way about a do-it-yourself clinic.

If you decide to use the court, don't go yourself—except the first time to give your assistant confidence. For one thing, your time is much too valuable. There are other reasons why it's best for your assistant to go in your stead. A defendant is less likely to blame her when he loses the case. Also, the judge, being only human, sees people in a relative way. The "rich" doctor against the struggling father of eight presents him with a moral problem quite aside from the merits of the case. But a slim, young assistant politely giving information opposite a hulking, unshaven, and spluttering deadbeat merely reinforces the merits of your case.

What if you go get a judgment and then can't find out where your debtor works? You can reassign the account to an agency. Now that you have a judgment, it won't have so much trouble collecting. Or, for a couple of dollars you can purchase a credit report, requesting a verified place of employment, and do it yourself. Or you can turn to the chapter on investigating by phone, and have your assistant start in.

Why bother with an agency if you're going to use small claims? Because it shouldn't be used as a substitute for collection agencies or other means of getting your bills paid. Just the time involved, if you used a small claims court on a wholesale basis, would put you in the collection business yourself, rather than in the profession you've chosen. But for cases that fall just below the agency's suit line, which is often set at $100 or higher, collecting through a small claims court can be a profitable and satisfying way of sweeping in the money you've earned.

Before using small claims court for the first time

Phone the court clerk before sending anyone down.
You'll be told precisely what's required, and so save an
extra trip. Your assistant should complete each claim and
take it to court in person—at least the first few times—so
that she can become friendly with the clerk and get help
in correcting any errors you may be making. After that,
she can arrange to file claims by mail and can keep a
supply of forms on hand. This will keep her trips to the
courthouse to a minimum.

Following is some basic information about small claims court aimed
at answering some of the questions that your assistant may ask. With this
background, she can make calls to your local small claims court and find
out exactly how to prepare your first small claims action.

What is a small claims court?

A court in which disputes involving less than $500 (different in some
states) are decided promptly and economically. The hearings are informal.
The person filing the claim is called the plaintiff; the person against
whom the claim is brought is called the defendant.

What kind of cases are heard there?

Consumers seek damages from stores for defective merchandise; creditors
sue on unpaid bills; tenants sue to recover security deposits from
landlords; people sue to recover damages for physical injuries and
property damage.

Who can bring an action?

Any person, business, or corporation can sue or be sued in a small claims
court. You don't need an attorney. In fact, attorneys aren't allowed to
represent you in a small claims court without permission from the judge.

What does it cost?

It varies between states, but usually it's not more than $10, depending
upon the amount of the claim. The only other cost is the service charge,
plus mileage, incurred by an officer when he serves the claim and notice
on the defendant. This varies according to the distance traveled to locate
the defendant.

How do you start an action?

Go to the small claims department of the courthouse in the county in which the defendant lives or can be served. The clerk will give you the proper forms and assist you in their preparation.

How does the defendant find out about your claim?

The claim and notice must be served on the defendant by a qualified person. You can't serve these papers yourself, and service cannot be made by mail. A sheriff or his designated deputy will serve the papers on any defendant living in his county.

What must the defendant do?

Within 10 days after receiving this notice, he may:

1. Pay the claim to the clerk of the court.
2. Demand a hearing.
3. In some states, demand a jury trial.
4. Ignore the notice.

If the defendant pays your claim, the clerk will forward the money to you. You don't recover your filing fees and service costs. If the defendant demands a hearing, the clerk will notify both of you of the time and place. If the defendant demands a jury trial, you'll be notified that you must file a formal complaint. In that case, you'll need an attorney and the case will proceed like any other district court case.

What if the defendant demands a hearing?

You, or your representative, must appear at the proper time and place. If you fail to appear, your claim will be dismissed. It may not be filed again. If the defendant believes he has a claim against you he can file a counterclaim at the time he requests a hearing. Each party should bring witnesses, statements, receipts, contracts, notes, dishonored checks, or any other evidence bearing on the claim. After questioning both parties and examining the evidence, the judge will make his decision.

What if the defendant fails to respond to the claim?

If he fails to respond within 10 days following receipt of the notice, you're entitled to a judgment. In many states, you must request this judgment in writing; in others, you appear in court on the date given and, if the defendant doesn't show, you receive judgment by default. Usually, the judgment will also include the costs you've sustained.

What happens after the judgment?

If you've received a judgment and the defendant refuses to pay, you may be able to have his car or other personal property seized, his wages or bank account garnisheed, or a lien put on his real property (real estate), by transcribing to circuit court. You must pay a small charge for using these methods of enforcing your judgment, but these costs are recoverable from the defendant.

What to take along when filing a suit

The name and address of the person you're suing, the amount, and brief statement about the nature of the claim—including the date the claim became due. (If it was a series of treatments, use the last date.)

You'll also be expected to pay the small claims fee when you file. You'll have to arrange, through the sheriff's office, for service of the claim on the defendant, and to pay the service fee and mileage charges.

13

Charge interest on unpaid fees?

"To be, or not to be ..."

The whole subject of charging interest on fees owed too long is controversial. Not only is there a soul-wrenching debate over the ethics of a doctor "making money on money," but it also puts you in the thickets and brambles of wondering whether (a) it actually pays to charge interest, (b) it antagonizes your patients, (c) it constitutes poor public relations for the profession, and (d) the bookkeeping alone costs more than the interest gained.

I believe that doctors fall into three categories: Those who are unshakeably against the idea on purely ethical grounds. Those who are on the fence but who wouldn't necessarily be averse if they could be shown that it's beneficial. And those who feel that charging interest is only good business, if an extension of time for payment is allowed.

Part of the problem is the confusion created by the A.M.A.'s stand in making an ethical judgment against interest charges, but not prohibiting the individual doctor from making his own choice. The problem was further confused in 1968 by passage of the truth-in-lending laws. Under Regulation Z, the Federal Reserve Board specifically named "doctors and dentists and other professional people and hospitals" among those included in the requirements of the act. That was enough for many doctors. They already considered themselves on shaky ground; the confusion engendered by this regulation resolved the problem for them. Setting aside their business instincts, they opted for being ethically right. Still, before making a final decision, perhaps it wouldn't hurt to check out the advantages and disadvantages to see, just for the record, that the path through the minefield of Regulation Z is not necessarily as complex as some suppose.

As for the ethics of charging interest, it could be that the aversion shown by the older gentlemen on the A.M.A. Judicial Council is a throwback to an earlier age when doctors accepted chickens and home-canned goods in payment for their services, sat up nights with sick patients, knew their people intimately from birth to death, and made house calls.

Those days have passed. Doctoring is now a legitimate business. People generally realize that times have changed. You provide them with service to the best of your training and ability, charge for it, and expect to be paid. If they don't pay when the bill comes due, it costs you money to carry them on the books. That's where the interest comes in. Credit is a commodity in the marketplace, and it has a price. It's never free. Try to finance something yourself and find out. Educated people understand this and expect to pay for it. So there's no logical reason not to charge a reasonable price for credit when **you** grant it. Nevertheless, you may still choose not to charge interest—for purely practical reasons.

Let's say you decide to add interest as an incentive to get people to pay more promptly. Will it work? The answer, according to the doctors and clinics polled by Medical Economics, is "Yes" and "No." It works well on people who are money-conscious and watch their pennies. Such people, however, are most often credit-conscious as well, so they're not your problem.

Those who habitually pay late, or not at all, don't give a darn whether you charge interest or not. Their modus operandi is to spend their money as fast as they get it, and when they want something they buy it, regardless of price or carrying charges. Oh, if they get into a discussion with you about their unpaid bill, and you've charged interest on it, they're quite likely to throw this up to you as the reason they didn't pay in the first place. Don't you believe it. Charging interest has absolutely no effect on the paying habits of these people.

The remainder of your slow-pays are those who just don't have the money. These are the poor, and they traditionally pay a higher price for everything they buy. They usually can't pay you any faster no matter how much interest you pile on them, so interest charged as a stimulant has no effect.

In total, you'll find your accounts receivable going down after you impose interest, mainly as a result of prompter payment by the money-conscious. And you'll find your monthly income somewhat increased as a result of the interest you collect. The questions then become: If you decide to begin charging interest, how do you set it up? And how do you get around that dragon, Regulation Z?

Letter to patients

This letter forewarns patients that you plan to begin adding interest if their accounts become overdue. Get a supply of letters printed initially, then include one in each statement for two months prior to making the change. Send copies to other active patients, except those with a record of prompt payment.

Dear Patient:

On the advice of our C.P.A., we plan to include interest on all overdue accounts. The purpose is to help defray the costs we incur each month in handling such accounts.

Therefore, effective November 1, 1974, a FINANCE CHARGE of 1 PER CENT will be added each month to every account that is more than 30 days past due. This represents an ANNUAL PERCENTAGE RATE of 12 PER CENT.

Very truly yours,

Be sure that the capitalized letters are included in your version of the letter and that you use print of at least this same size. This is necessary in order to comply with the specifications of Regulation Z. Follow-up statements, after the date the interest charge becomes effective, should show:

Balance due	$100.00
FINANCE CHARGE at 1%	1.00
(ANNUAL PERCENTAGE RATE 12%)	_____
Total balance now due	$101.00

If you're using a billing service, there's really no problem. Simply tell them to add interest to your accounts and when you wish to begin. Have them notify your patients of the change in advance, and in writing, so that those who don't wish to pay interest can make other arrangements. (See the accompanying example of a suitable letter. It includes enough information to comply with the requirements of Regulation Z.)

Decide whether interest should be added to all your accounts—except those on which insurance has been billed but not yet received—beginning after the first month they become due, or after being past due for 30, 60, or 90 days. Probably the simplest and most effective way (and most profitable) is to begin charging interest after 30 days. For accounts already on your books when you begin charging interest, don't go back to day one. Simply add interest as if the account were just 30 days old.

If you use an outside billing system, all you need do is call in the representative and lay out what you want. He'll take it from there. If the billing is done in your office, it's still not much more difficult, once you've won over your office staff to the idea. This is particularly true if you use the rate of 1 per cent because it's so easy to figure. No chart is needed. To save unnecessary typing, have your statements printed, or have a rubber stamp made to use on each statement:

Previous balance carried forward	$
Less your payment	$ _____
Subtotal	$
FINANCE CHARGE of 1% per month (ANNUAL PERCENTAGE RATE 12%)	$ _____
Total balance now due	$

Some of the interest you'll never collect, because quite a few patients will pay the balance promptly without including the interest. Your assistant should be instructed to write off these small balances while she's also posting the payments, to avoid rebilling for the interest only—an expensive practice that won't earn you any money.

Suppose you decide not to charge interest on your accounts? If you make a practice of extending credit, you still come under Regulation Z.

This seems ridiculous if you're not making any charge for your credit, but it's true. Whenever your extension of credit exceeds four payments, you're bound by Regulation Z, which means that your statements must reflect the fact that you're charging NO interest:

Original statement

For professional services	$300.00
FINANCE CHARGE	NONE
ANNUAL PERCENTAGE RATE	NONE
Date finance charge applies	Not Applicable
Number of installments	Eight (8)
Amount per installment	$ 37.50
Installment due date	1st each month
Total payments	$300.00
Default charge	NONE
Security	NONE
Penalty charge	NONE
Refund of finance charge	Not Applicable

Follow-up billing

Balance due	$262.50
ANNUAL PERCENTAGE RATE	NONE
Date or period for payment to avoid penalty	Not Applicable

There are quite legal ways to get around Regulation Z. Just don't make any front-end financial arrangements, and mail a statement to each patient and accept whatever payment comes in. Or simply telephone the patient and suggest some financial arrangement. That's all many doctors do.

There's another way, though, because the wording of the law reads that it applies only to formal arrangements involving more than four payments. So make no formal arrangements for more than four monthly payments. This can really work to your advantage, as many clinics have discovered. They use Regulation Z as an excuse when explaining to patients why they just can't accept any payment arrangement requiring more than four payments.

On the other hand, if a patient says that he'll be paying $20 a month for eight months, that's perfectly acceptable. It doesn't fall under Regulation Z because it's not legally binding on both parties.

The addition of interest is an individual matter. It's being done successfully. It reduces accounts receivable by getting some of the money in sooner. It doesn't cause trauma among patients. But so far, despite all these plus factors, it's not being utilized by most doctors.

Assigning interest-carrying accounts to agencies

When assigning accounts to agencies, be sure to show clearly the amount of the balance that represents interest.

Agencies generally add interest to all accounts assigned to them and usually figure it back to the first date of charge. If they don't know that part of your bill represents interest, they'll unwittingly double the interest charged. Should it come up later—in court, for instance—you'll bear the blame.

Many agencies routinely don't split interest collected with their clients. Many doctors know this and don't care. But half the interest, which may be substantial in large bills of long duration, would certainly help defray costs that the patient has forced you to incur. This is also true in court actions that an agency may handle for you. The judge, in most instances, will allow interest at the legal rate to be included in the sum he rules must be paid by the defendant. There's no reason why at least half of it shouldn't be forwarded to the doctor.

Your best bet is to read carefully any contract or assignment that an agency has you sign, and cross out and initial any reference to its retention of all interest. Then, if you notice that its monthly checks to you include no interest, have a showdown on the issue.

14

Health insurance claims: Part I

"HIC and COB"

Once upon a time, every one of the more than 800 private insurance companies now active in the health-care field had its own individually designed claim form. The double squeeze—more and more patients being covered by insurance, plus the lack of uniformity among claim forms—bewildered, confused, overworked, and frustrated the doctor's assistant. For the insurance industry, the resulting frequency of errors— leading to prolonged corrective correspondence and delayed payments— meant increased costs and angry subscribers.

By 1955 more than 100,000,000 Americans were covered by health insurance, and a clerical crisis threatened.

The need for a standard but simple-to-fill-out claim form was obvious. The Health Insurance Association, through its Health Insurance Council, established the Uniform Forms Committee to try.

The problem was to devise a form that would work as a common denominator among the 800-plus insurance companies—a difficult task because the companies are competitive. Each has to offer a product that's either more appealing or less expensive than the others. To do that and still survive requires a juggling of the risks to be covered and the benefits to be paid.

The result is that every company offers a slightly different package, each containing its individual combination of deductibles, exclusions, exceptions, pre-existing condition rules, and specific benefits. A standard form would have to be flexible enough to encompass all those variations and still remain simple.

The job wasn't accomplished overnight. In fact, a significant number of smaller companies have not yet converted to the standardized form. But by 1973, the Health Insurance Council could report that more than 90 per cent of all claims were being filed on the standardized form.

To accomplish that minor miracle, the committee accumulated and reviewed the various items of information each company needed to process medical, surgical, and loss-of-income insurance claims. A list of questions was then assembled, and it was concluded that if these questions were answered, most claims could be processed by most companies most of the time. The list, arranged in a standard sequence and format, became the all-purpose Attending Physician's Statement for Health Insurance Claims—Group or Individual, commonly called Comb-1.

The form, of course, was a compromise. Just as a factory suit is purposely cut more loosely to fit more people than a tailor-made suit, so the standard form contains more questions than may be necessary for any single insurance company's needs.

The council then began a two-pronged approach to promote acceptance of the form among physicians and the insurance industry. In this it had the full cooperation of the A.M.A.

Physicians, wanting an all-purpose form to stock in their offices for insured patients who came in without forms, were asked to adopt the Comb-1 without any changes. (See Appendix.) The insurance companies were asked to participate by converting to the approved form, but in their version of Comb-1 to include only the questions they actually needed from those provided by the council. The companies were specifically requested not to add any questions of their own. In Form 2, which is a claim for individual rather than group insurance, questions 8, 9, 10, and 11 were left out, because they relate to disability and aren't needed by the company.

Without question, the insurance industry had to make a great sacrifice in terms of internal regrouping and retraining to adapt to these forms. The physicians' need to train assistants to handle the previous wide variety of forms has been greatly relieved. As a result, forms are prepared more easily, less correspondence is required, fewer assistants' hours are required to do the job, payment checks come in earlier, and friction with patients about delayed insurance checks has diminished.

Nevertheless, there has been some criticism of the form by the medical profession. Many of the questions are considered to be "investigative," "unnecessary," or "answerable by the patient." Perhaps they seem that way sometimes, but it must be remembered that a great deal of time and effort was put into this project by insurance experts and members of the A.M.A., working together to ensure that only the most necessary, reasonable, and understandable questions were adopted.

The insurance industry is quick to point out that insurance laws **prohibit** the paying of benefits to which insured persons are not entitled, and that insurance companies are obligated to administer claims in strict compliance with the contractual provisions of their policies.

Even if this were not so, the unavoidable laws of economics come into play. Insurance premiums are based on statistical risks. Without reliable information on such matters as whether a policyholder collecting disability benefits is able to return to work, the statistics change tremendously. Much larger premiums are required to assume the risk.

The trouble, then, is that a great many employers and individuals would be inclined to settle for smaller benefits rather than pay those larger premiums. As a result, that portion owed to you by the patient and not covered by insurance would increase, and inevitably your collections would suffer.

This same argument applies to what the industry calls "coordination of benefits." You and I might think of it as the case of patients whose health is insured by more than one insurance. Many people do have that these days, either because both husband and wife work and so are covered by two groups, or because they maintain a private insurance or two in an effort to hedge against rising medical expense. At first glance, it seems to present a moral problem.

After all, we think, they pay the premiums in good faith, why shouldn't insurance companies pay dual benefits when a claim is filed?

For the answer, we need to look at the economics of the situation. Group premium rates are competitive items. In calculating them as low as possible, the statistical assumption that some members of the group will be covered under more than one insurance is taken into account. So included in the policy is a "coordination of benefits" provision, abbreviated to "COB."

It works this way: When two companies have the coordination clause, they'll work together and pay all of the sick or injured patient's expenses. However, when two insurances are involved, and only one has the coordination of benefits clause in its policy, the insurer without the clause becomes the primary insurer. It will pay to the limit of its coverage first, then the other company will pick up the remainder of the bill.

In reality, and over the long haul, this works to everyone's advantage because it keeps premium costs down. Obviously, when benefits are paid in excess of expenses, neither the patient nor the doctor has a financial incentive to control the use or the cost of medical services. As a result, medical expense goes up; premiums for insurance go up.

As for standardized forms, increasing Government involvement still burdens the medical office with too many different forms to handle efficiently. Help, though, is just over the horizon. The A.M.A. has appointed a special committee to develop a "Universal Attending Physician's Billing and Third-Party Report Form." The purpose is to produce a form that can be used nationally and satisfy the requirements of any and all third-party payers. In addition to being a real boon to the individual doctor's office, this universal form can be used to fulfill the requirements of medical service bureaus as they become more and more involved in billing third-party payers for you, utilizing EDP. What's more, the form will be designed so that it can be used to bill patients directly.

From the evidence, we can safely conclude that the Health Insurance Council and the A.M.A. are working steadily and in close cooperation to reduce the burden of paperwork in the doctor's office.

Much of what you had reason to complain about in the past is disappearing. Can the same be said for the insurance companies? How satisfied are they with the cooperation they're getting from doctors?

To get the answer, I contacted some 800 companies. In the next chapter, we'll examine what they have to say about you.

15
Health insurance claims: Part II

"Sins of omission"

The rallying cry of all doctors and their assistants everywhere is: "Let's have less paperwork and less delay in receiving payment." If insurance companies had a rallying cry, it would be: "Let's have less paperwork and less delay in being able to make payments!" Does that surprise you? It shouldn't. Delays in processing and extra handling of claims double or triple their work and skyrocket their expenses.

After almost 20 years of working with doctors and their assistants, I was solidly in your camp. Blame lay not on the head of the overworked assistant, but on that of the recalcitrant insurance company. That was how I felt before my research for this book. Now I'm a little wiser, and I realize that the problem isn't really one of malice or incompetence on either side, but just an inability to visualize the situation from the other side's point of view.

Here's how the insurance people see it: At least three out of four of those who wrote to me emphasized incompleteness and a lack of legibility as among their biggest headaches. Too often, one or more of the 12 or 13 questions included in the attending physician's statement are left blank.

You or your assistants may feel that certain questions don't apply in a particular case. But the claims adjuster in the insurance office may have a rule book stating that those questions must be answered before he can authorize payment. So he must either send the claim back, or write to you for more information. Either way means delay.

Illegible handwriting is a headache for everyone who has to handle completed insurance claims. More time is wasted in trying to decipher hastily scrawled information than for any other reason. Here's a quote from one of the largest insurers of health care in the country:

> "It will be most helpful if you will stress as often and as strongly as possible the need for physicians and their assistants to be sure that forms are filled out legibly and completely. It is astonishing how often the patient's name is misspelled or given incompletely, and the doctor identified by a scrawled signature or 'hen track' that defies translation."

As so very many insurance companies pointed out: When it's impossible to read a doctor's signature on a claim, and in the absence of any other identifying information, a check just can't be made out to him. They strongly recommended that your name be typed in prior to your signing.

The next largest trouble area is the disability section of the Comb-1 form—questions 8 and 9. A big part of the problem is the habit some assistants have of filling in both questions, like this:

> 8. Patient was continuously totally disabled (unable to work)
>   From 1-12-72   Thru 1-26-72
>
> 9. Patient was partially disabled
>   From 1-12-72   Thru 1-26-72

Since the patient's policy may pay him while he's totally disabled, but not when he is partially disabled (with variations), such duplicate answers make the form impossible to process.

Your part of the problem is to decide what to fill in when you know that your decision will make a significant financial difference to an economically deprived family. The insurance company wants you to report the truth. Yet your honest answer, when it denies the patient benefits, may very well antagonize him to the point where he refuses to pay your bill.

The insurance company can't possibly make the decision without your help. The insured isn't entitled to benefits for which he's not eligible. You have no right to give the company's money away out of sympathy for a patient who's not insured. This remains one more of the unpleasant, but necessary duties that every physician must face at times.

The next two most commonly unanswered questions on Comb-1 are 4 and 5: **Date symptoms first appeared or accident happened,** and **Date patient first consulted you for this condition.**

Perhaps your assistant sometimes omits this information because she doesn't have it—you having failed to enter it on the chart. Since

How well do you handle insurance claims?

<table>
<tr><td></td><td></td><td>Yes</td><td>No</td></tr>
<tr><td>1.</td><td>My insurance claims are completed on a daily or, at most, a weekly basis.</td><td>☐</td><td>☐</td></tr>
<tr><td>2.</td><td>When I sign forms, my name has already been typed in by my assistant.</td><td>☐</td><td>☐</td></tr>
<tr><td>3.</td><td>I usually glance at the forms to be sure my assistant has filled in every blank.</td><td>☐</td><td>☐</td></tr>
<tr><td>4.</td><td>All my claims are typed, rather than handwritten.</td><td>☐</td><td>☐</td></tr>
<tr><td>5.</td><td>We maintain a supply of blank Comb-1 forms as a backup, but we always insist that the patient bring in the proper claim form if he wants us to bill his insurer.</td><td>☐</td><td>☐</td></tr>
<tr><td>6.</td><td>My assistant is instructed not to accept a claim form for processing until the patient has completed his part.</td><td>☐</td><td>☐</td></tr>
<tr><td>7.</td><td>A stock question that I invariably ask each patient, for medical as well as insurance purposes, is when he first became aware of his illness. I note this on the chart.</td><td>☐</td><td>☐</td></tr>
<tr><td>8.</td><td>It's my office policy for all forms to be filled out with unbiased accuracy—for our protection as well as for the patient's.</td><td>☐</td><td>☐</td></tr>
</table>

Total

absence of this information will surely delay your fee up to two extra weeks, it pays to cultivate the habit of entering it.

Another way to avoid unnecessary delay is to instruct your assistant **always** to make sure the patient has filled out his part of the form. Sometimes, you may be providing much more information than necessary and blaming the companies for their excessive demands. The companies say that's because you're using your own blank Comb-1 forms (which include all 13 questions) instead of each company's version, which requires less information. Try to get the patient to give you the right form.

After all that, you may be wondering how your office stacks up. To find out, fill in the short quiz above. If all your answers are Yes, you can be sure that no doctor gets paid more promptly than you. Up to four Nos, you could be causing some of the delay; with a little tightening up you could boost your take-home pay within a few months. More than four Nos, you really need to review your insurance procedures. Even if the delay in receiving payment doesn't bother you too much, the errors your office is making are causing much needless work. Beyond that, your patients are probably needlessly worrying about the insurance payment that just doesn't arrive.

Aside from this smoothing out of procedures—which would help you as much as the insurance companies—it's good to bear in mind that the insurance industry and the medical profession share parallel interests. The insurance companies are just as appalled as you by the soaring cost of medical care. They view the increasing clamor for total Government intervention in the health-care field with apprehension.

They believe that everyone, rich or poor, should have access to quality health care. But they also believe that delivering and financing this care should remain within the province of private enterprise. They would like to see all Americans covered for all health-care needs, including: hospitalization, convalescent care, home health care, visits to the doctor's office, baby care, inpatient doctor services, and unlimited outpatient examinations and laboratory services. They want this both from the moral point of view and, quite frankly, because it would be good business. Very few physicians would disagree.

16

Health insurance claims: Part III

"Oh, how I hate to ..."

At least half of your doctor's income is received from insurance companies. So next time you sit down to complete a stack of claims, don't say, "I think I hate this part of the job worst of all." Instead think, "This must be the second most important job in this office."

It really is important, and you can do much to change it from a confusing, boring, do-it-later job into an example of competence that your doctor can be proud of. Then, when other doctors mention what a mess their own insurance desk is, he can say, "Insurance? No problem. Sandy stays right on top of it."

Fortunately, certain fairly simple procedures can cut the insurance job down to size. This chapter is designed to help you by answering any questions about the basic problems. Although approaches may vary according to type of practice and other circumstances, the rules that follow will apply to most offices and you'll find most of the problems they cover quite familiar. Check to see which rules you're already following and which may help streamline your procedures:

1. One week is a reasonable time after treatment in which to have filled in and mailed out insurance forms.
2. Save typing time on forms by using a rubber stamp of your doctor's name, address, and phone number.
3. Always try to use the standard HIC form. When a patient brings

another type of form, complete the HIC and staple it to the other. If the other form contains a question that's not on your HIC, be sure to answer it; otherwise you'll probably have your form returned for the missing information and end up handling it twice.

4. When an insurance company asks for information that's not on its own form, the best procedure is to reply that it must secure a release from the patient.

5. The most important source of information for completing the attending physician's statement is the doctor.

6. Five weeks is a reasonable time to wait before reminding the insurance company of an unpaid claim.

7. When an insurance company is slow in paying a claim, and the doctor instructs you to follow up, adopt a pleasant tone in your call or letter because that gets the best results.

8. Keep a copy of all claims you complete, particularly for workmen's compensation. Then, if a claim is lost, you can easily reproduce it. Occasionally, on workmen's compensation cases, your doctor may need it to handle a dispute over the bill. It's a lot easier to come up with a copy than to try to reconstruct the original from memory.

9. All treatment information, such as size of wound, number of stitches, bone fractures, time involved in treatment, etc., must be completed carefully on the form because it will influence the size of the doctor's fee and may save you the trouble of answering a request from the insurer for more information.

10. Disability information, either complete or partial, must be completed without ambiguity. Precise information is required on most policies before payment can be authorized.

Checklist for completing insurance claims

DID YOU: Spell the patient's name correctly?

Include all charges?

Fill in the policy or group numbers correctly, if required?

Get the prognosis from the doctor, if required?

Put a dash in each space that you didn't need to fill in?

Type in or rubber-stamp your doctor's name?

Make sure the authorization to release information is signed?

Make sure that the assignment of benefits is signed?

Make sure that the patient completed his part?

Keep a copy?

Your insurance logbook

Recommended procedure for any doctor's office is to keep an insurance logbook of some sort. It's the only way to know where you stand. The logbook should show the patient's name, insurance company or plan, policy number, date he presented his form, and the date it was mailed to the insurer.

Additional notes may give a history of the claim, including any missing information, inquiries made, or problems encountered in processing. You can see from the example that follows how much more efficient such a log is than notes on scraps of paper or hasty jottings on the patient's ledger. A logbook also serves as a quick check on outstanding claims. Just put a red check in the remarks section whenever a claim is paid. In that way, as you flip through the book, an overdue claim becomes very obvious. Set a time each week for checking your log and following up on overdue claims.

Let's suppose that you've correctly completed and sent in the forms, waited the suggested five weeks, and still no check has come in. What should you do?

If the company is local, call and tell the claims department of the insurance company that you filed a claim five weeks ago and have received nothing. Give the patient's name, policy or group number, your doctor's name, and your name and phone number. Get the name of the person you talk to and ask to be called back, today. If the company isn't local, send a follow-up form letter. (See page 103.) Enter the date in your log and mark your calendar for a second follow-up in 10 days.

Insurance claims log

Patient's name & Policy #	Insurance Company	Date in	Date out	Insurance Payment Received	Remarks

Follow-up letter to insurance company

Name and address
of insurance company   Date

Re: Insured's name:
    Patient's name:
    Policy #:
    Group #:

Gentlemen:
    More than five weeks ago we submitted a claim form
to you on behalf of your above-named insured. We have
received neither check nor rejection notice from you.
    A copy of the original claim is enclosed. May we hear
from you by return mail?

                             Very truly yours,

(Including a photocopy of the claim eliminates extra delay should the
insurer reply it has no record of the claim and request another copy.)

In at least one respect, contacting an insurance company is like all
the other business contacts you'll make throughout your life: It pays
to know someone in the company. Nothing beats the personal touch in
getting red tape set aside and putting your claim at the head of the list
to be paid.

All doctors' offices have perhaps a dozen companies with which they
file most claims. They're the ones in which you should cultivate your
contacts. Begin by calling and asking the name of the assistant manager
of the claims department. If it's an out-of-town company, get your
doctor's O.K. to make your first contact by phone. Explain that you'll
use mail once you have a name to write to. Address all correspondence
to this person. If he's local, and you telephone, always insist on speaking
with him. Be friendly and understanding; he has problems too. If you're
pleasant about it, he'll usually find your claim and see that it gets
processed. When you get the check, make a point of thanking him for
his helpfulness.

Keep your contact list in front of your logbook of insurance claims.
Then, in your absence, the contacts will be available to your replacement.

"Pay as you go" is the most practical and satisfactory way for a
patient to take care of his doctor bill. But if you don't know how much
the insurance covers and you want to give the patient credit for it, you're

likely to find yourself waiting for the insurance payment before you send the bill, thus denying your doctor use of the money he has earned.

The efficient assistant keeps tabs on the types of insurance claims she receives most frequently. She knows the allowances for the surgery and treatment covered by her doctor's specialty. She gives the patient credit for this amount only, and requires payment as he goes for the remainder. This keeps the accounts receivable low. It also eliminates a lot of collection problems on older bills.

One other thing you must do, however, is to keep a patient informed about the status of his claim if it's in any way out of the ordinary. When an insurance company questions any coverage, make a copy of the letter and send it to the patient. Keep him informed. If he doesn't hear from you for five or six months, and suddenly you tell him his claim has been rejected, he's going to feel that it's your fault. Tell him the minute a claim is overdue or becomes suspect. He'll get after the insurance company, too, and may even push the claim through for you.

To cut down your paperwork, it's best to have a standard letter to send patients:

> Dear Patient:
> This is to keep you informed about the progress of your insurance claim. As you know, we filed it for you right after you gave it to us. Now it is _____
> We _____ suggest that you get in touch with your _____ to see if there is anything you can do to expedite matters.
>
> Very truly yours,

In the first blank you would write in: **overdue, being investigated,** or **returned for more information.** In the second blank, write **do** or **do not.** In the third, you might put: **union, personnel department,** or **insurance company,** whichever is applicable.

Quite often patients will bring in their forms or even their insurance policies, and ask you to help determine the extent of their coverage. There's an advantage in knowing a patient's coverage; it provides a better idea of how much credit to extend on the strength of the insurance. But if the questions are too complicated, it's best to refer them to their insurance agent, union, or personnel manager.

In any case, a working knowledge of the terminology and basic types of insurance will help you figure out the claims you process and determine patients' benefits. Some of the terms and procedures we're about to mention may not be applicable to your doctor's practice. In other cases you may feel the need for more detailed information. This

104

you can easily get by calling your new contact at one of the insurance companies you deal with most.

Major types of health insurance

Nonprofit plans

The best known are Blue Cross and Blue Shield. Blue Cross pays for specific hospital services covered by each plan. Blue Shield helps pay doctor's fees for medical and surgical services. It pays participating doctors directly.

Commercial plans

These policies are purchased from commercial insurance companies by patients or their employers. They vary widely in coverage and usually give the patient the option of payment of benefits to him or to his doctor.

Prepayment plans

These are often sponsored and subsidized by employers or unions, although a growing number are being organized and run by groups of doctors. The patient receives care from participating physicians by paying an annual fee for total coverage.

Government-sponsored plans

A growing amount of medical coverage is now being provided by Government agencies, or by carriers operating under Government regulation and control. Programs and coverage change frequently, so you'll have to be on your toes and keep up to date. You'll be concerned mainly with these programs:

Medicare. There are two parts in this Federal program for patients 65 or over. (All dollar figures discussed in this Medicare section are for 1974, and are subject to change.)

Part A, hospital coverage, is financed by Social Security contributions from people while they work, with matching contributions from employers. Most persons 65 or over are entitled to coverage, but they must enroll in the plan during specified periods. The patient must pay the first $84 of hospital costs each year.

Part B, medical and surgical coverage, is presently voluntary. The insured must apply within a specified time and pay a $6.70 monthly premium. Matching contributions come from the Federal Government. If a patient says he's covered by Medicare, ask for his identification card, which shows whether he's covered only under Part A, or under both Parts A and B.

Medicare pays for the doctor's services under Part B coverage in one of two ways. In the assignment method, payment is made by the Medicare carrier directly to the doctor. When the doctor "accepts assignment," he agrees to let the carrier determine a reasonable and customary fee for each procedure, and to accept that amount for his full charge. The patient is responsible for the first $60 of charges in each year, plus 20 per cent of the eligible charges beyond that $60 deductible. Medicare pays the remaining 80 per cent. When there's a difference between the amount a doctor normally bills for a procedure and the amount Medicare determines to be reasonable, the doctor may not bill the patient for the difference.

If your doctor accepts Medicare assignments, you'll need to complete Part I of the Request for Medicare Payment form for each charge, and have it signed by the patient. After the patient has signed or completed Part I himself, complete Part II, have the doctor sign it, and forward it to the Medicare carrier. You'll also need to bill the patient for the first $60 of charges in each year.

When a doctor doesn't accept assignments, all fees are strictly between the doctor and the patient, and all Medicare payments are strictly between the patient and the Medicare carrier. If the doctor's statement itemizes and explains charges, the patient simply attaches the itemized statement to the Request for Medicare Payment form, completes and signs Part I, and sends it to the carrier. If the statement doesn't itemize charges, the patient completes and signs Part I, and returns the form to you. You complete Part II and return it to the patient, or forward it to the carrier. The carrier will pay the patient 80 per cent of what it determines to be a reasonable charge for the procedure, and the patient is responsible to the doctor for the entire bill.

Medicaid. This is a plan sponsored by both Federal and state governments. Coverage and benefits vary widely from state to state, so you must get the details from local authorities. Individual doctors also are likely to have their own rules for handling Medicaid patients.

Workmen's Compensation. All states have workmen's compensation laws to protect workers against loss of wages and medical expenses resulting from occupational accidents or disease. The information that must be supplied by the doctor is usually extensive, and the requirements vary from state to state. Contact the state bureau that handles workmen's compensation for instructions and the proper forms. When you mail the forms, be sure to keep copies in case the matter goes up for review.

Military medical benefits. Since 1956, under the CHAMPUS program, dependents of military personnel, both active and retired, have been authorized to receive treatment from civilian physicians, with the Government bearing some of the expense. Outpatient-care benefits were added in 1966. There is a deductible each year ($50 for an individual, $100 for a family), and the Government's contribution toward the doctor's bill varies according to the status of the "sponsor," the military husband or father. A special Military Dependents Claim form, furnished and filled out by the patient, must be used.

Insurance plans

Do you know the difference between hospital, medical, surgical, and major-medical plans? And what about personal accident, liability, and indemnity plans? A thorough understanding of the various plans will help you do your job quickly and accurately. There are five major forms of health insurance: hospital, surgical, regular medical, major-medical, and disability:

Hospital plans pay for hospital room and board, and some special services, such as X-rays. **Surgical plans** cover all or part of surgical expense. **Medical plans** cover nonsurgical physician's fees. **Major-Medical policies** are designed to offset unusually heavy medical expenses resulting from prolonged illness or serious injury. **Disability Income Protection plans,** sometimes called loss of income protection, provide cash benefits to policyholders unable to work because of accident or illness.

Other forms of insurance include: **Personal Accident,** which generally makes lump-sum payments in case of accidental death and loss of sight or limbs. **Liability** provides benefits to an individual injured in or by the insured's auto, or in his home or place of business. **Life Insurance,** from which proceeds are sometimes used to meet the expense of the insured's last illness.

Another way of categorizing health insurance is by how benefits are paid: **Indemnity plans** pay a specific amount toward specified procedures or services, such as $200 for an appendectomy. **Service Benefit plans** pay for surgical or medical service under arrangements whereby the participating physician agrees to accept the allowed benefits as full payment—if the insured's income falls within specified limits. Since there's no set fee schedule under most of these plans, payment is very much influenced by the accuracy and details of the information you send.

Insurance terminology

There are many terms you must understand precisely in order to follow instructions in filling out forms. Here are some of the most common:

— *Assignment of insurance benefits.* Usually made part of the claim form. By signing this part, the patient authorizes his insurance company to pay the doctor directly.
— *Beneficiary.* The person or persons designated to receive a specified

cash payment upon the policyholder's accidental or natural death.

— *Claim.* A demand to the insurer by the insured for the payment of benefits under a policy.

— *Coinsurance.* A policy provision, frequently found in major-medical insurance, under which the insured and the insurer share hospital and medical expenses resulting from an injury or an illness, in a specified ratio.

— *Deductible.* A term used mainly in major-medical plans referring to the amount of covered expense that must be paid by the insured before his policy's benefits begin.

— *Disability.* A condition that renders an insured person incapable of performing one or more of the duties required of him by his regular occupation.

— *Effective date.* The date coverage takes effect. (Look out for a waiting period—an initial number of days during which no coverage is in force for illness that begins during that period.)

— *Eligible family members.* Usually the spouse and any unmarried children within specified age limits.

— *Exclusions and exceptions.* Specific illnesses, injuries, or conditions listed in the policy for which the insuring company will not pay.

— *Fee or benefit schedules.* Payments set by insurance companies, especially in indemnity policies, for each service or procedure.

— *Income limit.* Sometimes a policy is a service policy for any person whose income falls below a certain limit. The insured receives all benefits without additional charge if his doctor is participating.

— *Insuring clause.* A statement in a policy listing benefits and the circumstances in which they'll be paid.

— *Lapse.* Termination of a policy when the policyholder fails to pay premiums within the required time.

— *Other Benefits.* Specified in each policy. They include X-ray, laboratory charges, drugs, oxygen, blood.

— *Participating physician.* A doctor who has joined a group or enrolled with the insurance company and has agreed to accept the contracts.

— *Patient services.* Either "inpatient," which means admitted to the hospital, or "outpatient," which means a person who is receiving services at the hospital but not staying there.

— *Pre-existing condition.* A physical condition that existed prior to issuance of the insured's policy. Some companies don't cover them; others will pay only after a specified waiting period.

— *Premium.* The periodic payment required to keep an insurance policy in force.

— *Release of information.* If an insurance company requests more information than is contained in the forms you send, you must ask the company to secure a release from the patient. A signed

108

authorization is also needed for information that may be requested by an attorney or other third party.

— *Termination conversion.* The process by which an employe, after leaving a company, has his group policy converted to an individual policy.

As you've seen, insurance is a detailed and complex subject, and one that involves a lot of routine but important work. To keep from getting bogged down, try making some basic resolutions about how you'll handle claims. Consider these:

Resolved: Every form will be completed and mailed within a week after a service is rendered.

Resolved: I'll get the patient's basic insurance information on the first visit, noting the type of insurance, the group, code, and any certificate number on the patient's history record and account card.

Resolved: I'll send reminders to insurers who have not paid within five weeks from the time completed forms are mailed.

Resolved: If necessary, I'll even "bug" the doctor to get any information I need to do the best possible job for him.

17

Health insurance claims: Part IV

"Don't hold your breath"

An ancient proverb has it that "No matter how high you rail your fence, one goat will get over." And so it is with insurance claims. No matter how good a relationship you have with the companies, or how careful you are in your own operation, once in a while a claim will go in and you just won't get paid. You wait, send your inquiry letter, wait again, and still no word. Why don't they answer?

To find out what can happen, I toured the head office of an insurance company. Before I tell you what I learned, you should know that health insurance companies range all the way from shoe-box operations paying out just a few thousand dollars a year in benefits, to immense corporations spewing out hundreds of millions in benefits. And there's just as wide a range between the efficiency levels of the various claim offices. Most companies specialize in life insurance; their health and accident insurance is a secondary source of income.

Consider, for example, Prudential Life Insurance Company—large, well-known, highly respected. During 1970, its life insurance premiums topped $2,200,000,000. In contrast, its receipts from sales of health and accident plans produced $738,000,000, roughly one-third as much.

Scale those figures down to sums that smaller companies handle, and you can see why your medical claim may not be their top concern. Even in the larger companies, where the income justifies hiring the best help available, there's bound to be a desk or two where efficiency is less than desirable.

The claims department I toured was aswarm with people working against a vibrating background cacophony of calculators and typewriters. Claim forms were everywhere, but I was told that they moved along in orderly and fairly routine manner. Claims that apparently slow up the works by requiring special handling usually involve large amounts, doctors' fees out of line for the services rendered, and ineligible preconditions. The longest delays, however, are caused by claims without answers to one or more key questions. That's what really exasperates claim handlers. They tend to push such claims aside for later processing.

Usually, your claim will be handled by a single adjuster. And if you write asking the whereabouts of your check—and if you've identified your claim correctly—your letter will go to him. More often than not, claims aren't identified sufficiently to be easily picked out of the thousands being handled. That means it has to wait its turn until a clerk-identifier gets to it. Occasionally, the company gets a note stating: "I sent you a claim form for my patient, Ethel Smith, over a month ago now. Where is the check?" Lots of luck on that one! But if you use the form letter in Chapter 16, the adjuster will have no trouble in identifying your claim.

Still, there's always that occasional one that falls out of step with the orderly, alphabetical army of forms and gets misfiled. Then, when your letter of inquiry arrives, clerks try to match it up with a claim and fail because the claim isn't where it's supposed to be. Rather than say, "Gee, we're sorry; we can't find your claim anywhere," they'll put your letter aside and wait for the claim to show up.

If you've followed the procedure outlined earlier, you have already waited five weeks before sending your inquiry. Now you've waited another 10 days and still no check—not even the courtesy of an answer. You're being ignored, you think, and it makes you mad. So you take one of your high-leverage alternatives—of which you have several:

Advise the patient that since his insurance company apparently isn't paying the bill, you now look to **him** for full payment. This is effective, but very tough on the patient. And it could be misleading. It's better, we think, to ask him to straighten out the problem with the insurance company himself. Then, should you not hear from patient or company in 10 days, send him the bill.

A more drastic approach is to write the company stating your intention to refer the matter to the state insurance commissioner. If **that** letter doesn't get results, you really do have a problem, and the sooner you report it the better. This, however, is firing your biggest gun when you probably don't need to. A letter along the following lines, addressed to the president of the company, will get you the same results without getting you on his list of troublemakers:

Dear Sir:

On July 19 of this year I submitted the claim identified above to your company for processing. After five weeks, I followed up with a polite note requesting information.

My note has been ignored and, knowing that this could not be normal policy for your company, I am choosing to write to you personally rather than take one of the more serious steps that my attorney advises.

May I expect the courtesy of a prompt reply about the disposition of the claim?

Very truly yours,

Insurance companies are almost paranoiacally aware that their success is absolutely dependent on their reputation. Rare is the top-line executive who didn't come up through the sales ranks. When a successful salesman sells a policy, he invariably sells himself at the same time on the performance of his company. He believes in it and, unlike the clerk in his claims department, will be galvanized into action by your complaint. Your chances are very good that the missing claim will be searched out, processed, and the check mailed on that same day—by executive order.

If the problem is a check for an amount less than the patient's contract, a different approach will be more successful. Your wisest course is to tell the patient how much the company paid and ask him to pay the balance. Explain that it's a matter strictly between him and his insurance company to straighten out. If he tries and gets no satisfactory explanation, tell him to get his attorney to fight it out. The only exception to that advice would be when the insurance company advised the patient that the reduced check was related to the value of your services. In that case, turn to your medical society's insurance review committee and have it investigate.

Insurance companies, like doctors' offices, are managed by fallible people. With that in mind, here's a final word of advice: Before taking any action that may boomerang, take a long, hard look at your copy of the claim form. Claim forms have been known to arrive at insurance headquarters without the doctor's name on them. A moment's checking may save your face as well as your blood pressure.

18

Converting other claims to Comb-1

"Spreading the word"

Making the Comb-1 work for any medical claim form, no matter how quaintly worded or wildly investigative, is the very best way to stay on top of your claim form workload. That holds true whether you're new on the job and don't know your way around the various forms, or a longtime professional in the claims game.

If you're an old-timer, I can hear you saying now, "Oh yeah? I'll bet there's not a claim form in existence that I can't figure out—if you give me a few minutes." True enough. But at 3 P.M. some Friday, with your helper off on a long weekend and a dozen claim forms stacked up, even a couple of minutes saved on each form adds up. That extra half hour you save by using Comb-1s and not having to analyze strange forms may give you just enough time to finish and get them signed by the doctor before he leaves.

Some experts advise sending in the plain Comb-1 form on every claim you receive, and if the insurance companies don't like it they can lump it. For practical reasons, I can't agree. Your purpose in filling out claim forms is to get your doctor paid or patients reimbursed, so any action that may delay payment is contrary to the best interests of your doctor and his patients. Nevertheless, it would be to everyone's advantage if all companies converted to the Comb-1 form. For that reason, I recommend using the Comb-1 form in every case—to get them used to it—but also giving the additional information some companies want.

To make it possible for you to use the Comb-1 exclusively, I've devoted the final section of this book to a "quick reference" system for converting all forms to Comb-1. The tools you'll need to put the system to work are in the appendix following this chapter. They consist of (a) an index of insurance companies, (b) a category explanation sheet, (c) an "additional information" sheet, and (d) a set of individual claim forms. Here's how the system is designed to work:

The companies listed in the index pay 90 per cent of all private medical insurance benefits—a total of $9,000,000,000 a year. Companies not listed are typically small and keep their operations within one state. Once you've become familiar with the system, you'll be able to convert their forms to Comb-1, simply by analyzing the particular form and adding a page for that company in the appendix.

Every company listed has been grouped in one of five categories, according to the type of claim form it uses. Immediately following the list of companies, you'll find the category explanation sheet, giving the special instructions required to convert the claim forms in the various categories to Comb-1. For example: If you get a claim form from, say, Prudential Insurance Company, check the index for the category number —in this case, Roman numeral I. Turning to the instructions for Category I, you'll learn that Prudential will accept the Comb-1 as is.

Category II is almost as simple to handle. Categories III, IV, and V require use of the "additional information" sheet, but you should have no problems.

Category V consists of companies whose requirements are so varied that their claim forms can't be converted under one set of instructions. Therefore, each is presented separately, with its individual form and conversion requirements.

By using the extracted and grouped requirements of companies that aren't satisfied with Comb-1, you'll have no need to analyze their forms at all. Simply fill out Comb-1 the way you usually do and add the extra items four of the categories call for. To start with, I suggest that you have "additional information" sheets made up similar to the example in the appendix. Then, as you process each claim, follow this procedure:

1. Glance in the index to find the category number of the company. In most cases it will be I, which means that the company has settled for the Comb-1 alone. You need look no further.
2. For codes other than I, check the category explanation page for the additional questions you'll have to answer in order to get the claim paid. The exception is Code V. For that, turn to the special group of companies whose varied requirements had to be listed individually.
3. Fill out the Comb-1 as usual; include whatever other information is necessary on an "additional information" sheet, and staple it to the reverse side of the Comb-1.

That's all there is to it. You've satisfied the insurance company, used the Comb-1 that you're used to, and avoided struggling through unfamiliar special forms. Undoubtedly, the insurance company people will be less than overjoyed about your method, but they'll be relieved at not having to correspond back and forth to get the information they need. Your claim will be processed more quickly, and you won't have to bother with follow-up letters to see what's delaying payment.

Appendix

Index of Insurance Companies

V Citizens Home Ins Co Inc
I Coastal States Life Ins Co
I Colonial Life & Accident Ins Co
I Colonial Life Ins Co of America
I Colonial Penn Life Ins Co
I Columbian Mutual Life Ins Co
I Columbus Mutual Life Ins Co
I Combined American Ins Co
III Combined Ins Co of America
III Commonwealth Life & Accident Ins Co
I Commonwealth Life Ins Co
I Commonwealth Mutual Ins Co of America
I Confederation Life Ins Co
I Connecticut Commercial Travellers Mutual
I Connecticut General Life Ins Co
I Constitution Life Ins Co
III Consumers Life Ins Co
I Continental American Life Ins Co
I Continental Assurance Co
III Cotton States Ins Group
I Country Life Ins Co
II Croatian Fraternal Union of America
I Crown Life Ins Co
I Cuna Mutual Ins Co

I Dominion Life Assurance Co

III Early American Life Mutual Ins Co
III Educator & Executive Ins Co
III Educators Life Ins Co of America
I Educators Mutual Life Ins Co
I Empire State Mutual Life Ins Co
I Employers Life Ins Co
I Employers Life Ins Co of America
I Employers Life Ins Co of Wausau, WI

I Employers National Life Ins Co
I Equitable Life Assurance Society
I Equitable Life Ins Co of Canada
III Equitable Reserve Assn
IV Equity Educators Assurance Co
I Excelsior Life Ins Co

I Far West Assurance Group Inc
III Farm Bureau Life Ins Co
I Farmers & Bankers Life Ins Co
I Farmers & Traders Life Ins Co
V Farmers New World Life Ins Co
I Federal Kemper Life Ins Co
I Federal Life & Casualty Co
I Federal Life Ins Co (Mutual)
I Federal Mutual Ins Co
I Federated Life Ins Co
I Fidelity & Guarantee Life Ins Co
II Fidelity Mutual Life Ins Co
V Financial Security Life Assurance Co
I Firemans Fund American Life Ins Co
II First Pyramid Life Ins Co of America
I Founders Life Assurance Co of FL
III Founders Life Ins Co of Los Angeles
I Franklin Life Ins Co

I Gamble Alden Life Ins Co
V Garden State Life Ins Co
I General American Life Ins Co
I General Reassurance Corp
I General Reinsurance Corp
III George Washington Life Ins Co
I Georgia International Life Ins Co
III Globe Life & Accident Ins Co
I Globe Life Ins Co

I Gotham Life Ins Co of NY
IV Grand Pacific Life Ins Co Ltd
I Great American Reserve Ins Co
I Great Southern Life Ins Co
I Great-West Life Assurance Co
III GSM (Golden State Mutual) Life Ins Co
III Guarantee Mutual Life Co
V Guarantee Reserve Life Ins Co
III Guarantee Trust Life Ins Co
I Guardian Life Ins Co of America
III Guardsman Life Ins Co
I Gulf Life Ins Co

I Hanover Life Ins Co
I Hartford Life & Accident Ins Co
I Hartford Life Ins Co
I Hawaiian Life Ins Co Ltd
I Hearthstone Ins Co of MA
III Home Life Ins Co
I Horace Mann Life Ins Co

I Illinois Mutual Life & Casualty Co
I Illinois Travelling Mens Health Assn
I Imperial Life Assurance Co of Canada
III INA Life Ins Co of NY
I Independent Liberty Life Ins Co
III Independent Life & Accident Ins Co
I Independent Order of Foresters
I Indianapolis Life Ins Co
I Industrial Life Ins Co
I Integon Life Ins Co
V Integrity National Life Ins Co
V International General Ins Corp
I International Life Ins Co
III Inter-Ocean Ins Co

V Investors Ins Corp
I Investors Syndicate Life Ins & Annuity
I Iowa State Travellers Mutual Assurance Co
I ITT Hamilton Life Ins Co
I ITT Life Ins Co of NY

I J C Penney Life Ins Co
I Jefferson National Life Ins Co
I John Hancock Mutual Ins Co

I Kansas City Life Ins Co
III Kentucky Central Life Ins Co

I Lamar Life Ins Co
V Legal Security Life Ins Co
I Liberty Life Assurance Co
I Liberty Life Ins Co
I Liberty National Life Ins Co
I Life & Casualty Ins Co of TN
I Life Ins Co of CA
V Life Ins Co of FL
I Life Ins Co of GA
III Life Ins Co of the Southwest
I Life Ins Co of VA
I Life of Mid-America
III Lincoln American Life Ins Co
III Lincoln Liberty Life Ins Co
I Lincoln National Life Ins Co (Ft. Wayne, IN)
I Lincoln National Life Ins Co (New York)
V Locomotive Engineers Mutual Life Ins Assn
I London Guarantee & Accident Co
I London Life Ins Co
I Lone Star Life Ins Co
III Louisiana & Southern Life Ins Co
I Loyal Protective Life Ins Co

I Lumberman's Mutual Casualty Co
I Lutheran Brotherhood
I Lutheran Mutual Life Ins Co

I Maccabees Mutual Life Ins Co
I Maine Fidelity Life Ins Co
I Manchester Life Ins Co
I Manufacturers Life Ins Co
I Marquette Life Ins Co
III Massachusetts Casualty Ins Co
I Massachusetts General Life Ins Co
I Massachusetts Mutual Life Ins Co
I Metropolitan Life Ins Co
I MFA Life Ins Co
I Michigan Life Ins Co
I Mid-American Mutual Life Ins Co
I Mid-Continent Life Ins Co
I Midland Mutual Life Ins Co
I Midland National Life Ins Co
III Midwest Life Ins Co
III Mid-West National Life Ins Co of TN
V Mid-Western Life Ins Co
I Ministers Life & Casualty Union
I Minnesota Mutual Life Ins Co
I Minnesota Protective Assn
I Monarch Life Ins Co
I Montgomery Ward Life Ins Co
I Montreal Life Ins Co
I Monumental Life Ins Co
V Municipal Ins Co of America
I Mutual Benefit Life Ins Co
I Mutual Life Assurance Co of Canada
I Mutual Life Ins Co of NY
I Mutual of Omaha Ins Co
III Mutual Savings Life Ins Co

I Mutual Security Life Ins Co
I Mutual Service Life Ins Co

I National-Ben Franklin Ins Corp
II National Farmers Union Life Ins Co
I National Fidelity Life Ins Co
I National Heritage Life Ins Co
I National Life & Accident Ins Co
I National Life Assurance Co of Canada
I National Masonic Provident Assn
I National Reserve Life Ins Co
I National Standard Life Ins Co
I National Travellers Life Co
III National Trust Life Ins Co
III National Western Life Ins Co
I Nationwide Life Ins Co
I New England Mutual Life Ins Co
I New Jersey Life Ins Co
I New York Life Ins Co
I North American Accident Ins Co
I North American Assurance Society of VA Inc
I North American Co for Life & Health Ins
I North American Life & Casualty Co
I North American Reassurance Co
III North Coast Life Ins Co
I Northern Life Ins Co
I Northwestern Mutual Life Ins Co
I Northwestern National Life Ins Co
I Northwestern Security Life Ins Co

I Occidental Life Ins Co of CA
III Occidental Life Ins Co of NC
I Ohio Casualty Ins Co
III Ohio National Life Ins Co
III Ohio State Life Ins Co

III Old Equity Life Ins Co
I Old Line Life Ins Co of America
I Old Republic Life Ins Co
I Old Security Life Ins Co
I Olympia National Life Ins Co

I Pacific Fidelity Life Ins Co
III Pacific Guardian Life Ins Co Ltd
I Pacific Mutual Life Ins Co
I Palmetto State Life Ins Co
I Pan-American Life Ins Co
III Parliament Life Ins
I Patriot Life Ins Co
I Paul Revere Life Ins Co
I Peerless Ins Co
I Pekin Farmers Life Ins Co
III Peninsula Life Ins Co
I Penn Mutual Life Ins Co
I Pennsylvania Ins Co
III Peoples Home Life Ins Co of IN
I Peoples Life Ins Co
I Petroleum State Ins Co
I Philadelphia Life Ins Co
III Phoenix Mutual Life Ins Co
I Piedmont Life Ins Co
I Pilot Life Ins Co
I Pioneer American Ins Co
I Pioneer Mutual Life Ins Co
I Professional Ins Corp
V Protected Home Mutual Life Ins Co
I Protective Life Ins Co
V Provident American Ins Co
III Provident Indemnity Life Ins Co
I Provident Life & Accident Ins Co
I Provident Life & Casualty Ins Co

I Provident Mutual Life Ins Co
I Prudential Ins Co of America
I Puritan Life Ins Co
I Pyramid Life Ins Co

I Ranger National Life Ins Co
I Reliance Standard Life Ins Co
III Republic National Life Ins Co
I Reserve Life Ins Co
V Reserve National Ins Co

I Safeco Life Ins Co
II St. Paul Hospital & Casualty Co
I San Francisco Life Ins Co
II Seaboard Life Ins Co
I Seaboard Surety Co
I Security Benefit Life Ins Co
I Security Ins Co of Hartford
I Security Life & Accident Co
III Security Life Ins Co
I Security Mutual Life Ins Co
IV Security of America Life Ins Co
I Sentry Ins, A Mutual Co
I Shenandoah Life Ins Co
III Southern Heritage Life Ins Co
I Southern Life Ins Co
I Southland Life Ins Co
I Southwestern Life Ins Co
III Sovereign Life Ins Co
I Springfield Life Ins Co
V Standard Life & Accident Ins Co of CA
III State Life & Health Ins Co
I State Mutual Life Assurance Co of America
I Sun Life Assurance Co of Canada
I Sun Life Ins Co of America

III Sunset Life Ins Co of America

I Teachers Ins & Annuity Assn
I Tennessee Life Ins Co
III Teton National Ins Co
III Tidelands Life Ins Co
I Time Ins Co
I Transamerica Ins Co
III Transport Life Ins Co
I Travellers Ins Co

I Underwriters National Assurance Co
I Union Bankers Ins Co
I Union Central Life Ins Co
III Union Fidelity Life Ins Co
I Union Labor Life Ins Co
I Union Life Ins Co
III Union Mutual Life Ins Co
V United Fidelity Life Ins Co
III United Founders Life Ins Co
III United Life & Accident Ins Co
I United Pacific Life Ins Co

I United States Life Ins Co

I Valley Forge Life Ins Co

I Washington National Ins Co
III Washington Square Life Ins Co
I West Coast Life Ins Co
I Western Casualty & Surety Co
I Western Life Ins Co
III Western Mutual Life & Casualty Co
I Westland Life Ins Co
III William Penn Fraternal Assn
II Wilson National Life Ins Co
I Wisconsin Life Ins Co
I Wisconsin National Life Ins Co
I Woodmen Accident & Life Co
I Woodmen of the World Life Ins Society
V Workmen's Benefit Fund of the USA
III World Ins Co

I Zurich American Life Ins Co
I Zurich Life Ins Co

The preceding list was compiled by direct contact with the insurance companies, and through the assistance of Richard Eales of the Health Insurance Council.

Category I
Every company included in the index with I after its name will accept the Comb-1 form (opposite) as approved by the Health Insurance Council.

Category II
These companies don't use a Comb-1 claim form, but all the questions on their own claim form are covered by the Comb-1. So you may confidently fill out the Comb-1, staple the company's form to the back of it, and send in both.

Category III
These companies have patterned their claim forms on an older version of the Health Insurance Council's recommendation. To satisfy them, you'll have to include:
1. Name and address of the hospital, if any used.
2. Date your doctor's services were terminated.
3. Whether an RN was required and used.

Use the Comb-1 and attach an "additional information" sheet, answering those three questions.

Category IV
This is a slightly more complicated Category III. You'll need the "additional information" sheet to include:
1. Name and address of the hospital, if any, and times entered and discharged.
2. Date your doctor's services were terminated.
3. Whether an RN was required and used.
4. Name and address of the referring doctor.

Category V
Each company in this category has different requirements that need separate instructions. The questions not covered by the Comb-1 have been listed for you opposite a copy of each company's individual claim form. Fill out the Comb-1, answer the questions listed on an "additional information" sheet—using the company's question numbers—and staple to the Comb-1.

Additional Information Sheet

Your question number:	Here is the additional information you requested on: _____ (insured)

ART A   TO BE COMPLETED BY PATIENT (INSURED)
Spaced for Typewriter - Marks for Tabulator Appear on this Line

TIENT'S NAME AND ADDRESS	DATE OF BIRTH

SURED'S NAME IF PATIENT IS A DEPENDENT

ME OF INSURANCE COMPANY	POLICY NUMBER	INSURED'S SOCIAL SECURITY NUMBER

GROUP INSURANCE, NAME OF POLICYHOLDER
e., Employer, Union or Association through whom insured)

THORIZATION TO PAY BENEFITS TO PHYSICIAN: I HEREBY AUTHORIZE YMENT DIRECTLY TO THE UNDERSIGNED PHYSICIAN OF THE SURGICAL D/OR MEDICAL BENEFITS, IF ANY, OTHERWISE PAYABLE TO ME FOR S SERVICES AS DESCRIBED BELOW BUT NOT TO EXCEED THE REASON- ILE AND CUSTOMARY CHARGE FOR THOSE SERVICES.

SIGNED (INSURED PERSON)

DATE

THORIZATION TO RELEASE INFORMATION: I HEREBY AUTHORIZE THE DERSIGNED PHYSICIAN TO RELEASE ANY INFORMATION ACQUIRED IN E COURSE OF MY EXAMINATION OR TREATMENT.

SIGNED (PATIENT, OR PARENT IF MINOR)

DATE

ART B   ATTENDING PHYSICIAN'S STATEMENT

DIAGNOSIS AND CONCURRENT CONDITIONS
(IF DIAGNOSIS CODE OTHER THAN ICDA* USED, GIVE NAME):

IS CONDITION DUE TO INJURY OR SICKNESS ARISING OUT OF PATIENT'S EMPLOYMENT? YES ☐ NO ☐   PREGNANCY? YES ☐ NO ☐   IF YES, APPROXIMATE DATE PREGNANCY COMMENCED. DATE

REPORT OF SERVICES (OR ATTACH ITEMIZED BILL) (IF PREVIOUS FORM SUBMITTED TO THIS CARRIER, YOU NEED SHOW ONLY DATES AND SERVICES SINCE LAST REPORT)

DATE OF SERVICES	PLACE OF SERVICES†	DESCRIPTION OF SURGICAL OR MEDICAL SERVICES RENDERED	PROCEDURE CODE - IF USED (IF CODE OTHER THAN CPT** USED, GIVE NAME)	CHARGES

® †O - Doctor's Office   IH - Inpatient Hospital   NH - Nursing Home
   H - Patient's Home   OH - Outpatient Hospital   OL - Other Locations
   *ICDA - International Classification of Diseases
   **CPT - Current Procedural Terminology (current edition)

TOTAL CHARGES ▶ $_____

AMOUNT PAID ▶ $_____

BALANCE DUE ▶ $_____

4. DATE SYMPTOMS FIRST APPEARED OR ACCIDENT HAPPENED.

5. DATE PATIENT FIRST CONSULTED YOU FOR THIS CONDITION.

6. PATIENT EVER HAD SAME OR SIMILAR CONDITION ?
YES ☐   NO ☐   IF "YES" WHEN AND DESCRIBE:

7. PATIENT STILL UNDER YOUR CARE FOR THIS CONDITION?
YES ☐   NO ☐

8. PATIENT WAS CONTINUOUSLY TOTALLY DISABLED (UNABLE TO WORK).
FROM   THRU

9. PATIENT WAS PARTIALLY DISABLED
FROM   THRU

0. IF STILL DISABLED, DATE PATIENT SHOULD BE ABLE TO RETURN TO WORK.

11. PATIENT WAS HOUSE CONFINED.
FROM   THRU

2. DOES PATIENT HAVE OTHER HEALTH COVERAGE? YES ☐ NO ☐
IF "YES" PLEASE IDENTIFY

13. I DO NOT ACCEPT ASSIGNMENT. ☐

DATE	PHYSICIAN'S NAME (PRINT)	DEGREE	INDIVIDUAL PRACTITIONER'S -SS#
PHYSICIAN'S SIGNATURE		TELEPHONE	ALL OTHERS - EMPLOYER I. D. #

MUST BE FURNISHED UNDER AUTHORITY OF LAW

STREET ADDRESS	CITY OR TOWN	STATE OR PROVINCE	ZIP CODE

MEMORANDUM REGARDING DISPOSITION OF THIS FORM ON REVERSE SIDE   Approved by the Council on Medical Service, A.M.A. 2/70

ACCREDITED HOSPITAL AND LIFE INSURANCE COMPANY
2360 Hampton Ave., St. Louis, MO 63114

Complete the Comb-1 form and include the following as additional information. Use the question numbers shown so the company will know which of its questions you're answering. Be sure to provide an answer to every question, even if it's "No" or "None."

2. Name and address of referring physician.

5d. If illness, is it acute, chronic, or congenital?

5 f. Prognosis:

6b. Name and address of hospital, if any used.

10. For what other illnesses or injuries, and when, have you previously treated patient?

ATTENDING PHYSICIAN'S STATEMENT

Patient's Name_____ Age _____

1. Date patient first consulted you for this condition:
    _____

2. Name and address of referring physician:
    _____

3. Primary diagnosis:
    _____
    _____

    (a) Secondary diagnosis or complications:
    _____
    _____
    _____

4. (a) When did illness begin or accident occur?   A.M.
    _____ __19 _____ P.M.

5. (a) History and diagnosis of sickness or character and extent of injury.
    _____
    _____

    (b) Complications, if any.
    _____
    _____

    (c) Describe the present condition of patient or injured parts.
    _____
    _____

    (d) If illness, is it acute, chronic or congential?
    _____

    (e) If illness, when in your opinion was the disease contracted or begun?
    _____

    (f) Prognosis.
    _____

6. (a) Was hospitalization required? If so, give date.
    Yes or No_____From _____ 19 _____ To _____ 19 _____
    (b) Name and address of hospital.
    _____

7. (a) If surgical operation was performed, describe fully or enclose copy of operative report.
    _____

    (b) When, where, and by whom. (Hospital, your office, etc.)
    _____

8. Give dates you treated patient.
    (a) At the hospital.
    _____
    (b) At his home.
    _____
    (c) At your office.
    _____

9. (a) Give dates patient was necessarily disabled from work and totally disabled.
                                                A.M.   A.M.
    From_____ 19_____ P.M. To _____ 19_____ P.M.

10. For what other illnesses or injuries have you previously treated patient, and when?
    _____
    _____

11. To what other insurance company or association or Workmen's Compensation Carrier are you reporting this?
    _____

Date _____ 19_____ Signed _____ M.D.

Address _____

City _____ State _____ Zip Code_____

Telephone _____ Physician's IRS or Social Security No. _____
         Area Code   Number

ASSIGNMENT OF BENEFITS: I hereby authorize payments of any benefits due under the terms of this policy to:

Doctor's Name:_____

Doctor's Address:_____

_____
                   Signature of Policyholder

AMALGAMATED LABOR LIFE INSURANCE COMPANY
2800 N. Sheridan Rd., Chicago, IL 60657

Complete the Comb-1 form and include the following as additional information. Use the question numbers shown so the company will know which of its questions you're answering. Be sure to provide an answer to every question, even if it's "No" or "None."

14. Name of hospital, if any, and date and time of both admission and discharge.

15. Was patient registered as a bed-patient?

16. Was confinement in a ward, semi-private, or private room? State which.

17. If suturing was done, how many stitches?

18. Was it cutting? Date of operation?

19. Was the abdominal approach used?

20. List X-ray and lab work done.

21. Where was this performed?

22. Findings of diagnostic work.

ATTENDING PHYSICIAN'S REPORT

LEASE ASSIST YOUR PATIENT BY COMPLETING THIS FORM

atient's Name_____ Age____ Is this disability the result of: Sickness ☐ Injury ☐

PLEASE COMPLETE THIS SECTION IN ALL CASES

. Date patient first treated for present disability_____ At Office_____Home_____Hospital_____

. Diagnosis (In adequate detail)_____

. How long has the disease existed and what history given? _____

. In your opinion, is disability due to any injury or illness arising out of patient's employment? Yes ☐ No ☐

. If so, explain_____

. If disability is a result of pregnancy, give approximate date of conception_____19____

. Is this person under your personal care at present? Yes ☐ No ☐ If not, when discharged?_____

COMPLETE TO SHOW MEDICAL TREATMENTS

Dates which you have personally given treatment.   your charge per call

. Patient's home_____ $_____

. Your office_____ $_____

. Hospital _____ $_____

. Amount paid on above medical treatment charges $_____

COMPLETE ONLY IF PATIENT UNABLE TO WORK

. How long was patient of YOUR PERSONAL KNOWLEDGE continuously and wholly disabled by reason of this
  disability from attending to ANY PART of his/her work or business? From_____Thru_____19____

. This patient should be able to return to work on_____

COMPLETE ONLY IF HOSPITAIZED

. Entered_____ A.M. _____19____ left Hospital_____ A.M. _____19____
           Name of Hospital   P.M.   Date   P.M.   Date

. Was patient a registered bed patient? Yes ☐ No ☐

. Was confinement in a: Ward (three beds or more) ☐ Semi-Private room (two beds) ☐ Private room ☐

COMPLETE ONLY IF SURGERY WAS PERFORMED

. Nature of Operation_____

. If suturing, how many stitches_____

. Was it cutting? Yes ☐ No ☐   Date of
                                       Operation_____ Operation by Dr._____
. Was abdominal approach used? Yes ☐ No ☐   Amount Charged
                                       for Operation $_____Amount paid on this charge $_____

COMPLETE ONLY IF DIAGNOSTIC X-RAY OR LABORATORY SERVICES PERFORMED

List X-ray and laboratory work done_____
          or

. Where performed_____ Date_____charge $_____

. Findings _____ Amount paid on above charge $_____

. To your knowledge, does patient have other health insurance or health plan coverage? If "Yes" identify.
  Yes ☐ _____ No ☐

| Print or Type Doctor's Name | Date of Signing This Form | DOCTOR SIGN HERE |
| Telephone Number | Signature of Attending Doctor | |

ocial Security or Tax I.D. No.   Street, City and State of Doctor

ART IV.   ASSIGNMENT OF INSURANCE BENEFITS:

I hereby authorize payment directly to the above named doctor of the Group Surgical Benefit specified in
 doctor's bill and otherwise payable to me but not to exceed the surgical fee for this particular benefit. I under-
nd I am financially responsible to the doctor for charges not covered by this assignment.

te___ _____19____ Signed_____
                                                    Insured

AMERICAN HOSPITAL AND LIFE INSURANCE COMPANY and
AMERICAN SECURITY LIFE INSURANCE COMPANY
P.O. Box 2341, San Antonio, TX 78206

Complete the Comb-1 form and include the following as additional
information. Use the question numbers shown so the company will
know which of its questions you're answering. Be sure to provide an
answer to every question, even if it's "No" or "None."

8. Is patient still under your care for this condition?
   If discharged, show date.

9. If patient hospitalized, give name and address of hospital.
   Give date admitted and date discharged.

15. How does the patient presently spend his or her time?

16. Is the patient mentally competent to endorse checks and direct
    the use of the proceeds with a clear understanding of the nature
    of his or her acts?   Yes   No

AMERICAN HOSPITAL & LIFE INSURANCE COMPANY

ATTENDING PHYSICIAN'S STATEMENT
– ACCIDENT OR SICKNESS –

Patient's Name and Address   Age _____

Nature of sickness or injury.
(Describe complications, if any)

Is condition due to pregnancy?   Yes ☐ No ☐

When did symptoms first appear or accident happen?

Date _____, 19 _____

When did patient first consult you in person at your office or at his (her) home for this condition?

Date _____, 19 _____

Has patient ever had same or similar condition?
(If "yes", state when and describe)   Yes ☐ No ☐

Describe any other disease, infirmity or previous disability affecting present condition.

Nature of surgical or obstetrical procedure, if any.
(Describe fully)

Give dates of treatment.

Office _____

Home _____

Hospital _____

Is patient still under your care for this condition?
If discharged, give date.   Yes ☐ No ☐

Date _____, 19 _____

9. If patient hospitalized, give name and address of hospital.

	Hospital	City	State
Date Admitted _____, 19 ___	Date Discharged _____, 19 ___		

10. How long was or will patient be continuously totally disabled (unable to work)?

From _____, 19 ___ through _____, 19 ___

11. How long was or will patient be partially disabled? (Disabled from performing a substantial part, but not all of his (her) important daily duties)

From _____, 19 ___ through _____, 19 ___

12. Was patient confined to the house?   Yes ☐ No ☐
(If "yes", give dates)

From _____, 19 ___ through _____, 19 ___

13. When was or will patient be able to resume any part of his (her) work?

Date _____, 19 _____

14. Is condition due to injury or sickness arising out of patient's employment? Is it covered by Workmen's Compensation, Employers Liability Insurance or Occupational Disease Law? (If "yes", explain)   Yes ☐ No ☐

15. How does the patient presently spend his (her) time?

16. Is the patient mentally competent to endorse checks and direct the use of the proceeds with a clear understanding of the nature of his (her) acts?   Yes ☐ No ☐

REMARKS

ate _____, 19 _____

Signed _____ D.O.
(Attending Physician)   M.D.

Phone _____

(Street Address)   (City or Town)   (Zone)   (State or Province)

OTE – Please sign authorization on reverse side.)

TO BE COMPLETED BY THE EMPLOYER

Date employee last worked _____ ___, 19 _____
Totally disabled (unable to work)

From _____, 19 ___ to _____, 19 _____
Partially disabled (disabled from performing a substantial part, but not all of his (her) important daily duties)

From _____, 19 ___ to _____, 19 _____
Exact date returned to work full time

Date _____, 19 _____

Duties employee was unable to perform during partial disability

6. Was he full or part time employee at beginning of disability?

7. Is employee to resume work for your Company?

8. Is disability the result of occupational injury or occupational disease?

9. Has disability been reported to anyone as a Workmen's Compensation Claim?

ate _____, 19 _____

Signed _____

Name of Company

By _____

Name and Official Position

Address _____

26 (Rev. 2-64)

ASSOCIATED LIFE INSURANCE COMPANY
1 E. Wacker Dr., Chicago, IL 60601

Complete the Comb-1 form and include the following as additional information. Use the question numbers shown so the company will know which of its questions you're answering. Be sure to provide an answer to every question, even if it's "No" or "None."

5. Did patient previously have medical attention for this condition? When?   By whom?

8. If confined to hospital, give name of hospital.

11. Dates confined to hospital: Dates confined to home:

13. Are you the family physician? For what have you previously treated patient?   When?

14. Has patient any chronic or constitutional disease, physical defect, or deformity? Give details:

ASSOCIATED LIFE INSURANCE COMPANY

PHYSICIAN'S STATEMENT

tient_____Age_____

dress_____

| Street | City | Zone | State |

Your diagnosis

_____

Is condition due to

illness ☐   accident? ☐

Date disability occurred_____

Date you were first consulted for this disability_____

Previous disability_____

Did patient previously have medical attention for this condition?
Yes ☐   No ☐

Date _____

By whom_____

His address_____

If illness, how long prior to your first examination was disease contracted or begun?

Years_____ Months_____ .Weeks_____

Is this illness a primary condition?
Yes ☐   No ☐

If not, what other disease is it secondary to, complicated with, or a sequence of?

_____

_____

If confined to hospital, give name of hospital

_____

9. Dates you treated patient for this condition   Charge Per Call

At office_____ _ _ $_____

At home_____ $_____

At hospital_____ $_____

10.. What operation was performed?

_____

Date_____Fee $_____ _____

11. Dates confined to hospital

From_____ To_____ .

Dates confined to home

From_____ To_____

12. Dates patient was disabled from performing usual duties

Totally from_____ to_____

Partially from_____ to_____

13. Are you the family physician?   Yes ☐   No ☐

For what have you previously treated patient?

_____

When? _____

14. Has patient any chronic or constitutional disease, physical defect or deformity?   Yes ☐   No ☐

Give details:

_____

_____

_____

---

ate _____   Signed_____ , _____

(Please also sign authorization on reverse side)   Degree

orm 625-AH

| Street Address | City or Town | State |

BANKERS LIFE & CASUALTY COMPANY
4444 Lawrence Ave., Chicago, IL 60630

Complete the Comb-1 form and include the following as additional information. Use the question numbers shown so the company will know which of its questions you're answering. Be sure to provide an answer to every question, even if it's "No" or "None."

3. Any previous medical attention for this condition? If "Yes," give date, doctor's name and address.
4. If illness, date symptoms first noticed. By whom?
5. For what have you previously treated patient?   Dates:
6. If patient has any chronic or constitutional disease or deformity, please give diagnosis and date first noted.
9. Name of hospital?   Dates confined:

DOCTOR, PLEASE SIGN HERE AS WELL AS BELOW

AUTHORIZATION I hereby authorize BANKERS LIFE & CASUALTY CO., Chicago, or its representatives, to inspect all X-ray pictures, clinical records and to obtain full information including etiology, diagnosis and prognosis, or other data that may be in your possession or under your control, and to make copies of same or any portion thereof, pertaining to the disability of _____

a patient in your hospital from _____ to _____

Date _____ Signed **X** _____

(Attending Physician) Degree

- -

DOCTOR'S CLAIM REPORT
TO SPEED CLAIM SERVICE, PLEASE ANSWER ALL QUESTIONS

PATIENT'S NAME _____ AGE _____

ADDRESS _____

(Street) (City) (State) (Zip Code)

POLICY NUMBERS _____

---

1. Diagnosis _____

   Is this condition primary?   Yes ☐   No ☐

   If no, what is it secondary to? _____

2. Is this illness? ☐   Accident? ☐   Pregnancy? ☐

   Date first consulted for this condition _____

   If accident, date _____ On job? Yes ☐   No ☐

   If pregnancy, what was expected
   date of full term delivery? _____

3. Any previous medical attention for this condition?

   Yes ☐   No ☐

   If yes, date _____

   Doctor's name _____

   Address _____

4. If illness, date symptoms first noticed _____

   By whom? _____

5. For what have you previously treated patient?

   _____ Date _____

   _____ Date _____

   _____ Date _____

6. If patient has any chronic or constitutional disease, physical defect or deformity, please give

   Diagnosis _____

   Date first noted _____

7. What operation was performed for present condition?

   _____

   Date _____ Your fee $ _____

   Does fee include charge for calls?   Yes ☐   No ☐

8. Dates you treated patient for present condition

   Charge Per Call

   At Office _____

   _____ $ ____

   At Home _____

   _____ $ ____

   At Hospital _____

   _____ $ ____

   Total charge for calls $ _____

   Your other charges
   (must be listed separately from calls)

   Medicine $ _____

   Laboratory $ _____

   X-ray $ _____

9. Name of Hospital _____

   Confined from _____ to _____

10. **ALSO COMPLETE IF PATIENT HAS LOSS OF TIME INSURANCE**
    Date disabled from performing usual duties:

    Totally from _____ to _____

    Partially from _____ to _____

    Was patient confined to the home?   Yes ☐   No ☐

    If yes, give dates: From _____ to _____

    If still disabled when will he probably
    be able to resume duties? _____

Date _____ Signed **X** _____

(Please also sign authorization above)   (Degree)   (Social Security or Tax No.—Required under authority of law)

Address _____

(Street)   (City)   (State)   (Zip Code)

458N   **TO AVOID DELAY PLEASE ANSWER ALL QUESTIONS**

CERTIFIED LIFE INSURANCE COMPANY OF CALIFORNIA
14724 Ventura Blvd., Sherman Oaks, CA 91403

Complete the Comb-1 form and include the following as additional information. Use the question numbers shown so the company will know which of its questions you're answering. Be sure to provide an answer to every question, even if it's "No" or "None."

3. Was there any previous medical attention for this condition? If "Yes," give date, doctor's name and address.

4. If illness, what date were symptoms first noticed? By whom?

5. For what have you previously treated this patient?   Dates:

6. If patient has any chronic or constitutional disease, physical defect, or deformity, please give diagnosis and date first noticed.

9. Give name of hospital used and dates confined.
   From: To:

DOCTOR'S CLAIM REPORT
TO SPEED CLAIM SERVICE, PLEASE ANSWER ALL QUESTIONS

ATIENT'S NAME_____ _AGE_____. How long a patient?_____

DDRESS_____
                              (Street)   (City)   (Zone)   (State)

Diagnosis _____

Is this condition primary?   Yes ☐   No ☐

If no, what is it secondary to?_____

_____

Is this illness? ☐   Accident? ☐   Pregnancy? ☐

Date first consulted for any of above_____19___

If accident, date_____ On job? Yes ☐   No ☐

If yes, state name and address of Workmen's Compensation, State Disability Plan or other insurance company to whom you are reporting this claim_____

If pregnancy, what was expected date of full term delivery?_____

Any previous medical attention for this condition?

Yes ☐   No ☐   If yes, date_____

Doctor's name _____

Address _____

If illness, date symptoms first noticed_____

By whom?_____

For what have you previously treated patient?

_____ Date_____

_____ Date_____

_____ Date_____

If patient has any chronic or constitutional disease, physical defect or deformity, please give

Diagnosis _____

Date first noted_____

7. What operation was performed for present condition?

_____

Date_____ Your fee $_____

Does fee include charge for calls?   Yes ☐   No ☐

8. Dates you treated patient for present condition

Charge Per Call

At Office_____

_____ $_____

At Home _____

_____ $_____

At Hospital_____

_____ $_____

Total charge for calls $_____

Your other charges (must be listed separately from calls)

Medicine $_____

Laboratory $_____

X-ray $_____

9. Name of Hospital_____

Confined from_____ to_____

10. **ALSO COMPLETE IF PATIENT HAS LOSS OF TIME INSURANCE**
Date disabled from performing usual work?

Totally from_____ to_____

Partially from _____ to_____

Was patient confined to the home?   Yes ☐   No ☐

If yes, give dates: From_____ to_____

If still disabled when will patient be able to resume usual work?_____19___

ite_____ Signed **X**_____
                                    (Please also sign authorization above)   Degree

ddress_____
                    (Street)   (City)   (State)

L-601 (1-71)   **TO AVOID DELAY PLEASE ANSWER ALL QUESTIONS**

CITIZENS HOME INSURANCE COMPANY, INC.
2601 Floyd Ave., Richmond, VA 23201

Complete the Comb-1 form and include the following as additional information. Use the question numbers shown so the company will know which of its questions you're answering. Be sure to provide an answer to every question, even if it's "No" or "None."

4. If no operation was performed, will one be necessary?

5. If ACCIDENT, give date injury was received, state where the accident occurred, and describe the nature of the accident.

8. Give the name of the doctor consulted by or having treated the pa icnt prior to your attendance.

9. Is the patient's present disability due solely to this sickness or injury?

10. What constitutional disease, physical defects, or deformities does claimant have?

11. Please give the name of any other company to whom you have reported this disability.

HOSPITALIZATION CLAIM — PHYSICIAN'S REPORT
CITIZENS HOME INSURANCE COMPANY, INCORPORATED
Richmond, Virginia

Name of Insured..Policy No.............................. Debit No....................

Address ....Date Blank Given to Physician............................

Name of Hospital...

Date Admitted...Date Discharged..

PHYSICIAN'S REPORT

1. Name of claimant... Age ....

2. Cause of disability ....

   ....

3. Was an operation performed? Describe fully...

   ....

4. If operation was not performed, will one be necessary?...

5. ACCIDENT—Date injury was received?...

   Where did accident occur? ....

   State nature of accident in full...

6. SICKNESS—When did sickness begin?...Is it chronic?.........................

   How long has patient had symptoms of ailment causing disability? ....

   Has claimant had this or any related disease before?......................... When? ....

   Is sickness due to or caused by pregnancy?...Is it venereal?.................

7. When did you first attend claimant for this disability?.....................................For previous disability?...............

8. Name of doctor consulted by or having treated patient prior to your attendance.......................................

9. Is claimant's present disability due solely to this sickness or injury? ....

10. If any, what constitutional disease, physical defects, or deformities does claimant have?...............................

    ....

11. Please give name of any other Company to whom you have reported this disability..

12. Is this disability covered by Workmen's Compensation?...

13. Additional remarks? ....

    ....

I HEREBY CERTIFY that the statements and answers made to the foregoing questions are strictly and wholly true, to the best of my knowledge and belief.

Signed by ...., M. D.

Date..., 19........   Address...

FARMERS NEW WORLD LIFE INSURANCE COMPANY
Mercer Island, WA 98040

Complete the Comb-1 form and include the following as additional information. Designate the question number exactly as shown so the company will know which of its questions you're answering. Be sure to answer this question, even if it's "None."

(second part) 8.   Names and addresses of other doctors consulted for this disability.

ATTENDING PHYSICIAN'S STATEMENT

Approved by Council on Medical Service, AMA Dec. 1959

PATIENT'S NAME AND ADDRESS	AGE

(1) NATURE OF SICKNESS OR INJURY (Describe Complications if any)

IS CONDITION DUE TO INJURY OR SICKNESS ARISING OUT OF PATIENT'S EMPLOYMENT? ☐ NO ☐ YES   IF "YES" EXPLAIN

IS CONDITION DUE TO PREGNANCY? ☐ NO ☐ YES   IF "YES" WHAT WAS APPROXIMATE DATE OF COMMENCEMENT OF PREGNANCY? | DATE   19

(2) WHEN DID SYMPTOMS FIRST APPEAR OR ACCIDENT HAPPEN? | DATE   19

(3) WHEN DID PATIENT FIRST CONSULT YOU FOR THIS CONDITION? | DATE   19

(4) HAS PATIENT EVER HAD SAME OR SIMILAR CONDITION? ☐ NO ☐ YES   IF "YES" STATE WHEN AND DESCRIBE

(5) DESCRIBE ANY OTHER DISEASE OR INFIRMITY AFFECTING PRESENT CONDITION

(6) NATURE OF SURGICAL OR OBSTETRICAL PROCEDURE, IF ANY (Describe Fully)   C.R.V.S. NO. USED FOR THIS PROCEDURE

DATE PATIENT WAS PLACED ON MEDICATION FOR THIS CONDITION   DATES MEDICATION WAS RENEWED

CHARGE FOR THIS PROCEDURE $	DATE PERFORMED	WHERE PERFORMED	IF IN HOSPITAL: ☐ IN-PATIENT ☐ OUT-PATIENT

(7) GIVE DATES OF TREATMENTS | OFFICE_____   CHARGE PER CALL $_____
HOME_____   CHARGE PER CALL $
HOSPITAL   CHARGE PER CALL $

(8) WHAT OTHER SERVICES, IF ANY, DID YOU PROVIDE PATIENT?   ITEMIZE, GIVING DATES AND FEES
TOTAL CHARGES $

NAMES AND ADDRESSES OF OTHER DOCTORS CONSULTED BY THE PATIENT FOR THIS CONDITION:

(9) IS PATIENT STILL UNDER YOUR CARE FOR THIS CONDITION? ☐ NO ☐ YES

(10) HOW LONG WAS OR WILL PATIENT BE CONTINUALLY TOTALLY DISABLED (Unable to work)? FROM _____ 19 THROUGH _____ 19

(11) HOW LONG WAS OR WILL PATIENT BE PARTIALLY DISABLED? FROM _____ 19 THROUGH _____ 19

(12) DID TREATMENT REQUIRE HOUSE CONFINEMENT ☐ NO ☐ YES IF "YES" GIVE DATES FROM _____ 19 THROUGH _____ 19

REMARKS

Farmers New World Life Insurance Co. may examine patient's medical records upon presentation of authorization signed by the patient or a qualified person.

DATE   SIGNATURE (Attending Physician) PLEASE PRINT—THEN SIGN ABOVE YOUR PRINTED NAME   DEGREE

STREET ADDRESS	CITY OR TOWN	ZONE	STATE OR PROVINCE	Soc. Security # or Tax I.D. #

Claimant's Assignment (Read before signing)

TO BE COMPLETED AND SIGNED BY THE CLAIMANT FOR DIRECT PAYMENT TO HOSPITAL, SURGEON OR PHYSICIAN.
(This assignment may not be honored if signed by a dependent or person other than the claimant)

I hereby assign (Indicate which benefits are assigned)
☐ Hospital Expense Benefits to the Hospital
☐ Surgical Expense Benefits to the Surgeon
☐ Medical Expense Benefits to the Physician

Indicated hereon, to the extent of their interest established herein or by statements attached.

DATED... SIGNED..
(Signature of Insured Claimant)

FINANCIAL SECURITY LIFE ASSURANCE COMPANY
1600 W. 10th St., Little Rock, AR 72203

Complete the Comb-1 form and include the following as additional information. Use the question numbers shown so the company will know which of its questions you're answering. Be sure to provide an answer to every question, even if it's "No" or "None."

1. State present complaint in the patient's own words, including how, when, and where originated.

6. Is this condition due to, or the result of, any past illness or injury prior to this date? If "Yes," explain.

7. Have you treated patient for any other sickness or injury prior to this date? If "Yes," explain.

9. Does this patient have a tendency toward developing various types of illnesses?

11. If patient was hospitalized, show name and address of hospital.

12. If patient is no longer under your care for this condition, show date discharged.

13. Has this patient had previous medical attention for this condition? If "Yes," give date and doctor's name and address.

14. Does patient have any chronic or constitutional disease, physical defect, or deformity? If "Yes," please give diagnosis and date first noted.

FINANCIAL SECURITY LIFE ASSURANCE COMPANY

1600 West 10th Street   Little Rock, Arkansas

ATTENDING PHYSICIAN'S STATEMENT

PATIENT'S NAME	AGE	ADDRESS

STATE PRESENT COMPLAINT OR COMPLAINTS IN PATIENT'S OWN WORDS INCLUDING HOW, AND WHERE ORIGINATED. USE REVERSE SIDE UNDER 1-A IF MORE ROOM IS NEEDED.

YOUR DIAGNOSIS.

HAS PATIENT EVER HAD SAME CONDITION?	☐ YES ☐ NO WHEN?_____19____	HAS PATIENT EVER HAD SIMILAR CONDITION?	☐ YES ☐ NO WHEN?_____19____

IS CONDITION DUE TO PREGNANCY? ☐ YES ☐ NO   IF SO, WHAT WAS APPROX. DATE OF CONCEPTION?_____19____

WHEN DID SYMPTOMS FIRST APPEAR? _____19____   WHEN DID PATIENT FIRST CONSULT YOU FOR THIS CONDITION? _____19____

IS THIS CONDITION DUE TO OR THE RESULT OF ANY PAST ILLNESS OR ACCIDENT? ☐YES ☐NO   IF "YES", EXPLAIN ON REVERSE SIDE UNDER 6-B.

HAS PATIENT BEEN TREATED BY YOU FOR ANY OTHER SICKNESS OR INJURY PRIOR TO THIS DATE? IF "YES". STATE WHEN AND DESCRIBE.   ☐ YES ☐ NO

NATURE OF SURGICAL OR OBSTETRICAL PROCEDURE IF ANY. GIVE DATE AND DESCRIBE FULLY.

DOES THIS PATIENT SEEM TO HAVE A TENDENCY TOWARDS DEVELOPING VARIOUS TYPES OF ILLNESSES? ☐ YES ☐ NO

GIVE DATES OF YOUR TREATMENTS.	AT YOUR OFFICE	AT PATIENT'S HOME	AT HOSPITAL

IF PATIENT HOSPITALIZED, GIVE NAME AND ADDRESS OF HOSPITAL.

IS PATIENT STILL UNDER YOUR CARE FOR THIS CONDITION? ☐ YES ☐NO   IF "NO", GIVE DATE DISCHARGED _____19_____

HAS PATIENT HAD ANY PREVIOUS MEDICAL ATTENTION FOR THIS CONDITION? ☐YES ☐NO   IF "YES", GIVE DATE _____19____   DOCTOR'S NAME _____   ADDRESS _____

DOES PATIENT HAVE ANY CHRONIC OR CONSTITUTIONAL DISEASE, PHYSICAL DEFECT OR DEFORMITY? IF "YES", PLEASE GIVE.   DIAGNOSIS.   DATE FIRST NOTED.

PAST DISABILITY FOR THIS CONDITION. ☐ TOTAL FROM_____19___THROUGH_____19_____ ☐ PARTIAL FROM_____19___THROUGH_____19_____

ESTIMATED FUTURE DISABILITY FOR THIS CONDITION. ☐ TOTAL _____19____THROUGH_____19____ ☐ PARTIAL _____19____THROUGH_____19____

HAVE YOU FILLED OUT ANY OTHER CLAIM FORMS FOR THIS DISABILITY? ☐ YES ☐ NO   NAME_____ ADDRESS_____ NAME_____ ADDRESS_____

REMARKS:

SIGNED _____ DEGREE_____ DATE_____

ADDRESS_____
STREET ADDRESS   CITY   STATE   ZIP NO.

GARDEN STATE LIFE INSURANCE COMPANY
484 Central Ave., Newark, NJ 07102

Complete the Comb-1 form and include the following as additional information. Use the question numbers shown so the company will know which of its questions you're answering. Be sure to provide an answer to every question, even if it's "No" or "None."

3. Sex:

4. Occupation (if known):

5. History of occurrence as described by patient:

10. Is condition solely a result of this accident?
    If "No," explain:

12. Will injury result in permanent disfigurement or disability? If "Yes," describe:

16. Is patient still under your care for this condition?

ATTENDING PHYSICIAN'S REPORT

ATE	PATIENT'S NAME	ACCIDENT DATE	FILE NO.

HIS PHYSICIAN'S STATEMENT MUST BE COMPLETED BY THE ATTENDING PHYSICIAN BEFORE BENEFITS THAT MAY BE DUE HE PATIENT CAN BE DETERMINED. PLEASE RETURN THE COMPLETED FORM TO:

```
┌─              ┐  _____
                        CLAIMS DEPARTMENT



└_             ┘
```

PATIENT'S NAME AND ADDRESS

AGE	3. SEX	4. OCCUPATION (IF KNOWN)

HISTORY OF OCCURRENCE AS DESCRIBED BY PATIENT

DIAGNOSIS AND CONCURRENT OR CONTRIBUTING CONDITIONS *

WHEN DID SYMPTOMS FIRST APPEAR? DATE:	8. WHEN DID PATIENT FIRST CONSULT YOU FOR THIS CONDITION? DATE?

HAS PATIENT EVER HAD SAME OR SIMILAR CONDITION?
YES ☐ ☐ NO   If "YES" state when and describe*

IS CONDITION SOLELY A RESULT OF THIS ACCIDENT?
YES ☐ ☐ NO   If "NO", EXPLAIN *

IS CONDITION DUE TO INJURY OR SICKNESS ARISING OUT OF PATIENT'S EMPLOYMENT?
YES ☐ ☐ NO

WILL INJURY RESULT IN PERMANENT DISFIGUREMENT OR DISABILITY?
YES ☐ ☐ NO   If "YES", describe

PATIENT WAS DISABLED (Unable to work) FROM: THROUGH:	14. IF STILL DISABLED, DATE PATIENT SHOULD BE ABLE TO RETURN TO WORK:

REPORT OF SERVICES *

DATE OF SERVICE	PLACE OF SERVICE	DESCRIPTION OF SURGICAL OR MEDICAL SERVICE RENDERED	CHARGES
			$
			$
			$

TOTAL CHARGE TO DATE $

IS PATIENT STILL UNDER YOUR CARE FOR THIS CONDITION? YES ☐ ☐ NO	**ESTIMATED FUTURE CHARGES $**

DATE	PHYSICIAN'S NAME (Print)	PHYSICIAN'S SIGNATURE	IRS/TIN IDENTIFICATION NO

NO.	STREET	CITY OR TOWN	STATE	ZIP CODE

* Use Reverse Side If Additional Space Is Needed
-3-1172

GUARANTEE RESERVE LIFE INSURANCE COMPANY
128 State St., Hammond, IN 46320

Complete the Comb-1 form and include the following as additional information. Use the question number shown so the company will know which of its questions you're answering. Be sure to provide an answer to this question, even if it's "No."

14. Has patient consulted you for any other condition? If "Yes," state when and describe.

GUARANTEE RESERVE LIFE INSURANCE COMPANY

HAMMOND, INDIANA 46320

ATTENDING PHYSICIAN'S STATEMENT

1. Patient's name_____Age_____

2. AUTHORIZATION TO PAY BENEFITS TO PHYSICIAN: I hereby authorize payment directly to the undersigned Physician of the Surgical and/or Medical Benefits, if any, otherwise payable to me for his services as described below but not to exceed the reasonable and customary charge for these services.

  SIGNED (INSURED PERSON)

  _____

3. Diagnosis and concurrent conditions

4. Is condition due to injury or sickness arising out of patient's employment?   Pregnancy?   If yes, approximate date pregnancy commenced.

  Yes ☐ No ☐   Yes ☐ No ☐   Date

5. Report of services (or attach itemized bill) (If previous form submitted to this carrier, you need show only dates and services since last report)

Date of services	Place of services †	Description of surgical or medical services rendered	Procedure code - if used (If code other than CPT** used, give name)	Charges

O - Doctor's Office   IH - Impatient Hospital   NH - Nursing Home
H - Patient's Home   OH - Outpatient Hospital   OL - Other Locations
*ICDA - International Classification of Diseases
**CPT - Current Procedural Terminology (Current edition)

Total charges ▶ $_____
Amount paid ▶ $_____
Balance due ▶ $_____

6. Date symptoms first appeared or accident happened.   7. Date patient first consulted you for this condition.

8. Patient ever had same or similar condition?   9. Patient still under your care for this condition?
  Yes ☐ No ☐ If "yes," state when and describe.   Yes ☐ No ☐

10. Patient was continuously totally disabled (unable to work)   11. Patient was partially disabled.

  From   Thru   From   Thru

12. If still disabled, date patient should be able to return to work.   13. Patient was house confined.

  From   Thru

14. Has patient consulted you for any other condition Yes ☐ No ☐ (If yes, state when and describe _____

15. INDIVIDUAL PRACTITIONERS-SS#

  ALL OTHERS-EMPLOYER I.D.#
    must be furnished under authority of law   _____

Date_____Physician's name (print)_____

Physician's signature_____Degree_____Telephone_____

Street address_____City or town_____State or province_____ZIP code_____

INTEGRITY NATIONAL LIFE INSURANCE COMPANY
230 N. Thirteenth St., Philadelphia, PA 19101

Complete the Comb-1 form and include the following as additional information. Use the question number shown so the company will know which of its questions you're answering. Be sure to provide an answer to this question, even if it's "No."

3c.   If performed in hospital, give name of hospital.

INTEGRITY NATIONAL LIEE INSURANCE COMPANY

ATTENDING PHYSICIAN'S STATEMENT – HEALTH INSURANCE CLAIM – INCOME PROTECTION APSC

Spaced for Typewriter — Marks for Tabulator Appear on this Line

IENT'S NAME AND ADDRESS | AGE

URED'S NAME IF PATIENT IS A DEPENDENT

POLICY NUMBER

GROUP INSURANCE GIVE NAME OF POLICYHOLDER
, Employer, Union or Association through whom insured)

A) DIAGNOSIS AND CONCURRENT CONDITIONS
(IF FRACTURE OR DISLOCATION, DESCRIBE NATURE AND LOCATION)

) IS CONDITION DUE TO INJURY OR SICKNESS
ARISING OUT OF PATIENT'S EMPLOYMENT? IF "YES" EXPLAIN
YES☐ NO☐

) IS CONDITION DUE IF "YES" WHAT WAS APPROXIMATE DATE
TO PREGNANCY? OF COMMENCEMENT OF PREGNANCY?
YES☐ NO☐ DATE 19

A) WHEN DID SYMPTOMS FIRST APPEAR OR ACCIDENT HAPPEN? DATE.....................................19....

) WHEN DID PATIENT FIRST CONSULT YOU FOR THIS CONDITION? DATE.....................................19....

) HAS PATIENT EVER HAD SAME
OR SIMILAR CONDITION? IF "YES" STATE WHEN AND DESCRIBE
YES☐ NO☐

A) NATURE OF SURGICAL OR OBSTETRICAL
PROCEDURE, IF ANY (Describe Fully)

DATE PERFORMED ....19....

) CHARGE TO PATIENT FOR THIS PROCEDURE
$..............

) IF PERFORMED IN HOSPITAL, GIVE NAME OF HOSPITAL
INPATIENT☐ OUTPATIENT☐

) GIVE DATES OF OTHER MEDICAL (NON-SURGICAL)
TREATMENT, IF ANY
CHARGE PER CALL
OFFICE.......................................$..............
HOME...$..............
HOSPITAL.....................................$..............
TOTAL (NON-SURGICAL) CHARGES $..............

) IS PATIENT STILL UNDER YOUR CARE FOR THIS CONDITION?
IF "NO" GIVE DATE YOUR SERVICES TERMINATED
YES☐ NO☐ DATE 19

A) HOW LONG WAS OR WILL PATIENT BE CONTINUOUSLY
TOTALLY DISABLED (Unable to work)?
FROM...................19... THRU...................19...

) HOW LONG WAS OR WILL PATIENT BE PARTIALLY DISABLED?
FROM...................19... THRU...................19...

) WAS HOUSE CONFINEMENT NECESSARY? IF "YES" GIVE DATES
YES☐ NO☐ FROM 19 THRU 19

) TO YOUR KNOWLEDGE DOES PATIENT HAVE OTHER HEALTH
INSURANCE OR HEALTH PLAN COVERAGE? IF "YES" IDENTIFY
YES☐ NO☐

DATE | SIGNATURE (ATTENDING PHYSICIAN) | DEGREE | TELEPHONE

STREET ADDRESS | CITY OR TOWN | STATE OR PROVINCE | ZIP CODE

6-5

Approved by Council on Medical Service, AMA November 1964

INTERNATIONAL GENERAL INSURANCE CORPORATION
P.O. Box 3667, Milwaukee, WI 53217

Complete the Comb-1 form and include the following as additional information. Use the question numbers shown so the company will know which of its questions you're answering. Be sure to provide an answer to every question, even if it's "No" or "None."

5. Did patient previously have medical attention for this condition or a similar one? If "Yes," give date, by whom, and address.

8. If confined to hospital, give name and address.

11. Show dates entered and discharged from hospital.

13. Are you the family physician? For what have you previously treated this patient? When?

14. Has patient any chronic or constitutional disease, physical defect, or deformity? Give details.

PHYSICIAN'S STATEMENT

PATIENT:_____ AGE:_____ TELEPHONE:_____

ADDRESS:_____ CITY:_____ STATE:_____

1. Your diagnosis:_____

_____

2. Date disability occurred:_____

_____

3. Is condition due to:
   Illness ( )   Accident ( )

4. Date you were first consulted for
   this disability:_____

5. Did patient previously have medical
   attention for this condition or
   similar one?   Yes( )   No( )

   Date:_____

   By Whom:_____

   Address:_____

6. If illness, how long prior to your first
   examination was the disease
   contracted or begun?
   Years_____ Months_____ Weeks_____

7. Is this illness a primary condition?
   Yes( )   No( )
   If not, what other disease is it
   secondary to, complicated with, or
   a sequence of?_____

   _____

8. If confined to hospital, name of
   hospital:_____

   Address:_____

9. Dates treated patient for this condition:_____

   _____

10. What operation was performed:
    _____ Date_____

11. Dates confined to hospital:
    From_____ To_____
    Dates confined to home:
    From_____ To_____

12. Date patient was disabled from per-
    forming duties:
    Totally from_____ to_____
    Partially from_____ to_____

13. Are you the family physician?
    Yes( )   No( )   For what have you pre-
    viously treated patient?_____

    _____

    When?_____

14. Has patient any chronic or constitutional
    disease, physical defect or deformity?
    Yes( )   No( )   Give details:_____

    _____

    _____

    _____

15. Comments:_____

    _____

    _____

    _____

Date:_____   Signed:_____

Address:_____

      Street   City   State   Zip   Telephone

EMPLOYER'S STATEMENT

Employee by the name of _____ Occupation_____

was away from work entirely from _____ to _____

due to _____.

He was able to resume light duties on _____ and full duties on_____

Would he have been on lay off or down time
if not on disability   Yes( )   No( )

Dated_____

_____
              Name of Company

_____
       Name and Official Position

INVESTORS INSURANCE CORPORATION
P.O. Box 12025, Portland, OR 97212

Complete the Comb-1 form and include the following as additional information. Use the question numbers shown so the company will know which of its questions you're answering. Be sure to provide an answer to every question, even if it's "No" or "None."

3. How long have you known the patient professionally?

5. What is patient's chief complaint?

11. Has patient consulted any other physician for this problem? If so, give name(s).

Mail to: INVESTORS INSURANCE CORPORATION
P.O. Box 12025
Portland, Oregon 97212

ATTENDING PHYSICIAN'S REPORT - TO BE RETURNED BY THE PHYSICIAN

PLEASE NOTE

This report is designed to provide specific information which usually permits immediate evaluation of the Insurance Benefits under all types of Health Insurance issued by Investors Insurance Corporation. Omissions of pertinent information often cause delay and inconvenience to the doctor and patient. Please review report for clarity and completeness before mailing.

1. Patient's NAME _____ Stated Age _____

2. Past Medical History:

3. How long have you known Patient professionally?

4. When did patient first consult you for present condition?

5. Chief Complaint:

6. Date symptoms first appeared:

7. To what do you attribute origin? (Please include dates)

8. Has patient ever suffered from this or similar condition in the past? (Please give symptoms and dates)

9. Final Diagnosis (es)

10. Date of Diagnosis (es)

11. Has patient consulted any other physician for this problem? (If so, Please give names)

12. Is condition due to injury or sickness arising out of patient's employment?   If so, is it presumed to be covered by Workman's Compensation or Employer's Liability Law?

13. How long was or will patient be continuously totally disabled (unable to work)?_____ from _____ 19_____ to _____ 19_____.

14. How long was or will patient be partially disabled?   from_____ 19_____ to _____ 19_____.

15. If sickness, was patient confined to the   Yes ☐
house? (If "Yes", give dates)   No ☐ from _____ 19_____ to _____ 19_____

ATTENDING PHYSICIAN'S IRS No. _____
This information is required by law.

Date of Report _____ Signed _____

ATTENDING PHYSICIAN

LEGAL SECURITY LIFE INSURANCE COMPANY
P.O. Box 8476, Dallas, TX 75205

Complete the Comb-1 form and include the following as additional information. Use the question numbers shown so the company will know which of its questions you're answering. Be sure to provide an answer to every question, even if it's "No" or "None."

6. Has patient previously had medical attention for this condition? If so, please give date, doctor's name and address.

7. How long have you been the patient's doctor?

8. Please give any pertinent past medical history.

12. Has the patient had a chronic or constitutional disease or physical defect not otherwise named in this form? If so, please describe.

13. For what other conditions has patient been treated within the past five years?

14. To what other insurance companies is this claim being made?

OTE TO ATTENDING PHYSICIAN: If all the questions below are answered clearly and in detail further cor-
spondence with you will not be necessary; your valuable time will be saved, and prompt disposition of the
aim may be made.

Claim No. _____

PHYSICIAN'S STATEMENT

ame of patient _____ Age _____ Policy Number _____

Your diagnosis or diagnoses (please give all)
_____
_____
_____

What, in your opinion, is the underlying cause
of this condition? _____
_____

Is condition acute? _____ Chronic? _____
Recurrent? _____

Date you were FIRST consulted for this disability _____

Date of FIRST symptoms _____

Short summary of history of this condition, its
nature and origin _____
_____
_____
_____

Has patient previously had medical attention
for this condition? _____
If so, date _____
Physician _____
Address _____

How long have you been patient's doctor?
_____

Pertinent past history _____
_____
_____
_____

9. If accident, is injury the sole cause of this
disability? _____
Complications, if any _____

10. Dates you treated patient for this condition:
At home _____
At office _____
At hospital _____
Charge per visit _____

11. What operation performed? _____
_____
Charge made _____

12. Has patient any chronic or constitutional disease or physical defect not otherwise named
on this form? _____ If so,
please describe _____
_____

13. For what other conditions has patient been
treated within the past five years?
_____
_____
_____
_____

14. To what other insurance companies is this
claim being made? _____
_____
_____

15. Is claim being submitted to Workmen's Compensation? Yes _____ No _____

ereby authorize the hospital to which _____ was confined to furnish to
EGAL SECURITY LIFE INSURANCE COMPANY any information regarding said patient's health, including
l hospital, X-ray, laboratory and other records, and to permit any representative of said Company to personal-
examine such records and to make copies of all or any part thereof. A photocopy of this authorization shall
considered as valid as the original.

Internal Revenue Ruling (69.595) Section 6041 requires your Social Security or Tax
Identification Number be reported. ➤ _____

ate _____

furnishing this blank and investigating this claim,
e company shall not be held to admit the validity
any claim or to waive the breach of any condition
the policy or application receipt.

Signed _____
          Attending Physician   Degree

Address _____

City _____ State _____

LIFE INSURANCE COMPANY OF FLORIDA
7800 S.W. Red Road, South Miami, FL 33143

Complete the Comb-1 form and include the following as additional information. Use the question numbers shown so the company will know which of its questions you're answering. Be sure to provide an answer to every question, even if it's "No" or "None."

1. Primary Diagnosis(es):
   Secondary Diagnosis(es):
   Complications, if any:
2. Is this condition due to illness? Accident?
3. If accident, give details:
5. How long have you been patient's doctor?
6. Was patient referred by another doctor?
   Referring doctor's name & address:
7. Name of hospital:
   Address:
   Dates:
8. Place surgical procedure performed:

ATTENDING PHYSICIAN'S STATEMENTS

Patient's Name _____ Age _____

1. Primary Diagnosis(es) _____

   Secondary Diagnosis(es) _____

   Complications, if any: _____

2. Is this condition due to illness? _____ Accident? _____

3. If accident, give details: _____

   _____

4. Has patient ever had prior treatment for this condition? _____

   If so, give date and describe _____

5. How long have you been patient's doctor? _____

6. Was patient referred by another doctor? _____

   Referring doctor's name and address _____

7. Name of hospital _____

   Address _____

   Dates confined: FROM_____ TO _____

8. Nature of surgical procedure _____

   Charge for surgical procedure $_____

   Place performed _____ Date performed _____

9. Dates of medical treatment by you:
   Office   Home   Hospital

   _____   _____   _____

Date_____ SIGNED X _____

                            ADDRESS _____

- -

LOCOMOTIVE ENGINEERS MUTUAL LIFE & ACCIDENT INSURANCE ASSOCIATION
1026 B. of L. E. Building, Cleveland, OH 44114

Complete the Comb-1 form and include the following as additional information. Use the question numbers shown so the company will know which of its questions you're answering. Be sure to provide answers to both questions, even if they're "Never" and "None."

22. When and for what have you previously treated this patient?

23. What, if any, chronic or constitutional disease or physical defects does the patient have?

THE LOCOMOTIVE ENGINEERS MUTUAL LIFE AND ACCIDENT INSURANCE ASSOCIATION

1026 B. of L. E. BUILDING   CLEVELAND, OHIO 44114

CLAIMANT'S STATEMENT FOR HOSPITAL AND SURGICAL EXPENSE

Furnishing this blank does not indicate admission of liability on the part of the Association.   78

1] BLE Division No._____ Policy No._____ Dated_____19_____

2] Name of Claimant_____ 3] Birth Date_____

4] Address

5] Employer's Name and Address

6] Date Injured or Taken Ill   7] Date Ceased Work

8] If Accident, how did it happen?
Include time and place

9] Describe illness or injury

10] If illness, when were
you previously troubled
with this condition?

11] Full Name and address of attending physician.

12] Full Name and address of family physician.

13] Date first treated

14] Hospital: Name   From: A.M.-P.M.   19

Address   To: A.M.-P.M.   19

15]   Claimant's Signature_____

IMPORTANT NOTICE: Premiums on your Hospital policy must be paid for the month in which disability occurs.
To avoid delays in processing your claim - PLEASE ATTACH YOUR PREMIUM RECEIPT FOR THE CURRENT
MONTH to this claim or have your Insurance Collector certify to the payment of the current premium by signing the
certification below:-

This is to certify that premiums on the above claimant's policy have been paid in full for the month of

_____.

Date_____   _____
                                Insurance Collector BLE Div._____

PHYSICIAN'S STATEMENT

16] Patient's Name:

17] Diagnosis:

18] Complications, if any:

19] Date first consulted: 20] Date of onset:

21] Operation, if any:

22] When and for what have you
previously treated patient:

23] What, if any, chronic or constitutional
disease or physical defect does patient have?

24]   Attending physician's signature_____

MID-WESTERN LIFE INSURANCE COMPANY
P.O. Box 1429, Enid, OK 73701

Complete the Comb-1 form and include the following as additional information. Use the question numbers shown so the company will know which of its questions you're answering. Be sure to provide an answer to every question, even if it's "No" or "None."

10. When, in your opinion, did the patient first become aware of some symptom of the condition?

12. If hospitalized, name and address of hospital:

13. Date admitted:

14. Date discharged:

15. Names and addresses of other physicians who have treated patient for this illness or injury:

18. To what other companies are you reporting this loss?

OKLAHOMA STANDARD CLAIM FORM

APPROVED BY THE OKLAHOMA STATE MEDICAL ASSOCIATION AND THE ASSOCIATION OF HEALTH AND ACCIDENT INSURORS OF OKLAHOMA

MID-WESTERN LIFE INSURANCE COMPANY

ATTENDING PHYSICIAN'S STATEMENT

PATIENT'S NAME	2. ADDRESS	ZIP CODE	3. AGE

DIAGNOSIS (EXPLAIN COMPLICATIONS)

ADDITIONAL DIAGNOSES (CHRONIC DISEASE OF DEFECT FOUND DURING PRESENT TREATMENT)

DATE OF ONSET	7. DATE FIRST CONSULTED	8. DUE TO PREGNANCY ☐ YES ☐ NO	9. COMPENSATION CASE ☐ YES ☐ NO	10. WHEN, IN YOUR OPINION, DID THE PATIENT FIRST BECOME AWARE OF SOME SYMPTOM OF THIS CONDITION?

. SURGICAL OR OBSTETRICAL PROCEDURES (DESCRIBE)

. IF HOSPITALIZED, NAME AND ADDRESS OF HOSPITAL	13. DATE ADMITTED	14. DATE DISCHARGED

NAME AND ADDRESS OF OTHER PHYSICIANS WHO HAVE TREATED PATIENT FOR THIS ILLNESS OR INJURY	ZIP CODE

OMPLETE IF PATIENT HAS INDICATED
OSS OF TIME BENEFITS

6. TOTAL DISABILITY:

FROM_____ TO_____

7. PARTIAL DISABILITY:

FROM_____ TO_____

AUTHORIZATION TO PAY PHYSICIAN

I HEREBY AUTHORIZE PAYMENT DIRECTLY TO THE ATTENDING PHYSICIAN FOR THIS ILLNESS OR INJURY, OF THE PHYSICIAN'S OR SURGEON'S BENEFITS OTHERWISE PAYABLE TO ME, BUT NOT TO EXCEED MY INDEBTEDNESS TO SAID PHYSICIAN. I UNDERSTAND I AM FINANCIALLY RESPONSIBLE TO THE PHYSICIAN FOR CHARGES NOT COVERED BY THIS ASSIGNMENT.

DATE_____ SIGNED_____

(INSURED)

☐ IS
. THE HOSPITAL ☐ IS NOT AUTHORIZED TO FURNISH, WITH THE INSURED'S CONSENT, ANY INFORMATION REGARDING THIS CLAIM,
REQUESTED BY THE_____INSURANCE COMPANY

To what other companies or associations are you reporting this loss? _____

TE_____SIGNED_____

PHYSICIAN	DEGREE

DRESS_____

STREET	CITY AND STATE	ZIP CODE

NOTE TO PHYSICIAN: PLEASE SUBMIT YOUR ITEMIZED STATEMENT FOR THIS CLAIM. OKLAHOMA PHYSICIANS MAY USE OSMA FORM 102.

PHYSICIAN I. D. OR S. S. NO. _____

INSURED'S STATEMENT

TO BE COMPLETED PERSONALLY BY THE INSURED
YOUR DOCTOR OR HOSPITAL IS NOT RESPONSIBLE FOR COMPLETION

LICY NO. _____   CLAIM NO. _____

ME	AGE	ADDRESS	ZIP CODE

IF ACCIDENT: GIVE DATE	DESCRIBE HOW AND WHERE IT HAPPENED

IF SICKNESS: GIVE NATURE OF COMPLAINTS

DATE YOU FIRST NOTICED SYMPTOMS OR REALIZED YOU WERE GETTING SICK	4. DATE FIRST SAW A DOCTOR

HAVE YOU HAD SYMPTOMS OR TREATMENT FOR THIS SICKNESS BEFORE	6. WHEN?

MEDICAL TREATMENT RECEIVED DURING LAST TWO YEARS

(SICKNESS)	(DOCTOR)	(YEAR)

What other insurance (Hospital, Surgery, Accident and Sickness) have you?

AUTHORIZATION

I HEREBY AUTHORIZE ANY HOSPITAL OR PHYSICIAN TO FURNISH TO THE_____INSURANCE
PANY OR ITS REPRESENTATIVE OR PERMIT SAID INSURANCE COMPANY OR ITS REPRESENTATIVE TO REVIEW ANY INFORMATION REQUESTED WITH RESPECT TO ANY
NESS OR ACCIDENT, MEDICAL HISTORY OR COPIES OF HOSPITAL AND MEDICAL RECORDS. A PHOTOSTATIC COPY OF THIS AUTHORIZATION SHALL BE CONSIDERED AS
ID AS THE ORIGINAL. I DECLARE THE ABOVE ANSWERS AND STATEMENTS ARE TRUE AND CORRECT TO THE BEST OF MY KNOWLEDGE AND BELIEF.

TE_____SIGNED:_____

M 400 - REV 5-62

MUNICIPAL INSURANCE COMPANY OF AMERICA
721 Dundee Ave., Elgin, IL 60120

Complete the Comb-1 form and include the following as additional information. Use the question numbers shown so the company will know which of its questions you're answering. Be sure to provide an answer to every question, even if it's "No" or "None."

5a. If condition is due to sickness, how long, in your opinion, prior to your first examination, did the condition originate?

b. Is the condition due to accidental injury? If "Yes," explain.

8. Is patient still under your care for this condition? If discharged, give date.

9. Did patient previously have any medical attention for this condition? If "Yes," give date, doctor's name and address.

10. If patient was hospitalized, give name and address of hospital, and dates admitted and discharged.

THE MUNICIPAL INSURANCE COMPANY
OF AMERICA

1 Dundee Avenue

Elgin, Illinois 60120

TTENDING PHYSICIAN'S STATEMENT

tient's Name_____ Age_____

Nature of sickness or injury. (Describe complications if any)	
When did symptoms first appear or accident happen?	Date_____, 19_____
When did patient first consult you for this condition?	Date_____, 19_____
Has patient ever had same or similar condition? (If "yes", state when and describe)	Yes ☐ No ☐
A. IF SICKNESS, in your opinion how long prior to your first examination did the condition originate or begin?	Years_____ Months_____ Weeks_____
B. Is condition due to accidental injury? If "yes", explain.	Yes ☐ No ☐
Nature of Surgery, if any, and date performed.	Date_____, 19_____
Give dates of treatment.	Office_____
	Home_____
	Hospital_____
Is patient still under your care for this condition? If discharged, give date.	Yes ☐ No ☐
	Date_____, 19_____
Did patient previously have medical attention for this condition?	Yes ☐ No ☐
	Date_____, 19_____
	By whom_____
	His address_____
If patient was hospitalized, give name and address of hospital.	_____
	(Hospital) (City) (State)
	Date Admitted_____, 19__ Date Discharged_____, 19__
How long was or will patient be continuously totally disabled (unable to work)?	From_____, 19__ through_____, 19__
How long was or will patient be partially disabled?	From_____, 19__ through_____, 19__

ate _____ Tel. No. _____

Signature of Physician_____ M.D.
(Please Also Sign Authorization Below)

ddress_____
(Street Number)

_____
(City)   *(State)*

Signature of Physician_____ M.D.

L 19A 10-67

PROTECTED HOME MUTUAL LIFE INSURANCE COMPANY
30 E. State St., Sharon, PA 16146

Complete the Comb-1 form and include the following as additional information. Use the question numbers shown so the company will know which of its questions you're answering. Be sure to provide an answer to every question, even if it's "No" or "None."

2. Was patient referred to you by another physician? If so, please give his name and address.

5. In your professional opinion, how long has this condition been present?

6. How long has patient known of this condition?

9. If patient was confined, state where, including address and dates admitted and discharged.

11. Has patient any chronic or constitutional disease or physical defect? Give details.

ATTENDING PHYSICIAN'S STATEMENT

To be completed by Attending Physician and forwarded to

PROTECTED HOME MUTUAL
LIFE INSURANCE COMPANY
Home Office SHARON, PENNSYLVANIA 16146

EALTH INSURANCE CLAIM – INDIVIDUAL

ient's Name and Address	Date of Birth

On what date did you first attend patient for this condition?

Was patient referred to you by another physician ?
If so, please give name and address of referring physician.

Describe in full the illness or injury with complete diagnosis and treatment.

a. Contributing cause or conditions

If condition due to pregnancy, please give approximate date of commencement of pregnancy.

Has patient previously suffered from same or similar conditions ?   Yes ☐ No ☐

If "Yes" state when and describe

In your professional opinion, how long has this condition been present ?

How long has patient known of this condition ?

Date patient totally disabled from work ?

From _____ 19 ____ to _____ 19 ____

Dates patient partially disabled from work ?

From _____ 19 ____ to _____ 19 ____

Dates patient confined from

_____ 19 ____ to _____ 19 ____

Place _____ Address _____

Description of medical treatment, obstetrical or surgical procedures.

_____ Fee Charged $ _____

_____ Fee Charged $ _____

Has patient any chronic or constitutional disease or physical defect? _____ Give Details

Indicate non-surgical and non-obstetrical visits "O" Doctor's Office; "H" Patient's Home; "NH" Nursing Home; "OH" Out-Patient Hospital;
"IP" In-Patient Hospital; "OL" Other Location?

Month	1	2	3	4	5	6	7	8	9	10	11	12	13	14	15	16	17	18	19	20	21	22	23	24	25	26	27	28	29	30	31

To what other companies, including Workmen's Compensation, have you reported this claim?

e	Physician's Name (Print)	Signature	Degree	Telephone

eet Address	City or Town	State	Zip Code

parate assignment of benefits is being submitted, doctor must furnish Taxpayer Identification Number as required by the Internal Revenue Code
pace provided below. This information is required to be furnished under authority of law.

Doctor's Tax Number [_____]

PROVIDENT AMERICAN INSURANCE COMPANY
5744 L.B.J. Freeway, P.O. Box 30161, Dallas, TX 75230

Complete the Comb-1 form and include the following as additional
information. Use the question numbers shown so the company will
know which of its questions you're answering. Be sure to provide an
answer to every question, even if it's "No" or "None."

1. How long have you been the patient's doctor?
4. In your opinion, how long has the condition which caused the
   disability been present?
6. What history did the patient give, as to etiology and date of onset?
7. Is the disease chronic? Recurrent? Sub-acute? Acute?
8. What complications arose while confined?
9. What other disabilities were treated during this confinement?
11. Does the patient have Medicare coverage?
12. If so, was a private room required by you, for him?
13. Did you require the attendance of a Graduate Registered Nurse?
    If so, dates required?
15. Has patient any chronic or constitutional disease or physical defect?
    If so, please give diagnosis.
17. What other medical or surgical treatment has the patient received
    in the last five years? (Give date, nature of illness or injuries.)
18. To what other companies have you reported this claim?

PROVIDENT AMERICAN INSURANCE COMPANY

An Old Line Legal Reserve Stock Company

5744 L.B.J. Freeway • P. O. Box 30161 • Dallas, Texas 75230

ATTENDING PHYSICIAN'S STATEMENT

Dear Dr.:

This Company strives at all times to process claims with the information furnished on the first form sent us. However, it sometimes becomes necessary to ask the doctor to provide additional information needed to process a claim, especially when all of the questions are not answered on the first form.

We would appreciate it greatly, Doctor, if you will answer the following questions fully, so that it may not be necessary to write you again for additional information, and take up your most valuable time.

Claim No.

PATIENT'S NAME	PATIENT'S AGE	IF IN HOSPITAL, CHECK ONE SQUARE
		☐ IN PATIENT ☐ OUT PATIENT

1. How long have you been patient's doctor?_____

2. Date you first attended patient for this disability?_____

3. With what disease or injury did you find patient afflicted?_____

   (A) What was the etiology of the condition?_____

   (B) Date you released patient?_____

4. In you opinion how long had the condition which caused the disability been present?_____

5. Has the patient previously suffered from the same or similar condition? If so, when?_____

   (A) What was diagnosis at that time?_____

6. What history did patient give, as to the etiology and the date of onset?_____

7. Was the disease chronic?_____ Recurrent?_____ Sub acute?_____ Acute?_____

8. What complications arose while confined?_____

9. What other disabilities were treated during this confinement?_____

10. What operation, if any, was performed?_____

   (A) Date of Operation?_____ What charge was made?_____

   (B) What laboratory examination made? (Check which) Urine_____ Blood Count_____ Tissue_____ Spinal fluid_____ What other type of laboratory work was made? Please specify._____

11. Does patient have Medicare coverage?_____

12. If so, was a private room required by you for the treatment of the disability?_____

13. Did you require the attendance of a Graduate Registered Nurse?_____ If so, give dates required._____

14. Give dates of treatment: Charge per call

   Office_____ $_____

   Home_____ $_____

   Hospital_____ $_____

15. Has patient any chronic or constitutional disease or physical defect? If so, please give diagnosis._____

16. How long had the condition been present?_____

17. What other medical or surgical treatment has patient received in the past five years? (Give date, nature of illness or injuries)_____

18. To what other companies have you reported this claim?_____

Any hospital or any doctor is hereby authorized to furnish the Provident American Insurance Company or its representative any and all information, including history records, that may be deemed necessary by the Company, with the insured's consent.

Physician's Signature _____ Degree _____ Date _____

Address_____

1000 Rev. 7/70   Physician's S S #_____

RESERVE NATIONAL INSURANCE COMPANY
418 Northwest 5th, Oklahoma City, OK 73102

Complete the Comb-1 form and include the following as additional information. Use the question numbers shown so the company will know which of its questions you're answering. Be sure to provide an answer to every question, even if it's "None."

5. Additional diagnosis (chronic disease or defect found during present treatment).

10. When, in your opinion, did patient become aware of some symptom of this condition?

12. If hospitalized, give name and address of hospital.

13. Date patient was admitted.

14. Date patient was discharged.

15. Name and address of other physicians who have treated the patient for this illness or injury.

STANDARD CLAIM FORM

RESERVE NATIONAL INSURANCE COMPANY
418 Northwest 5th
Oklahoma City, Oklahoma 73102

ATTENDING PHYSICIAN'S REPORT

ATIENT'S NAME | 2. ADDRESS | 3. AGE

>IAGNOSIS (EXPLAIN COMPLICATIONS)

ADDITIONAL DIAGNOSES (CHRONIC DISEASE OR DEFECT FOUND DURING PRESENT TREATMENT)

>ATE OF ONSET | 7. DATE FIRST CONSULTED | 8. DUE TO PREGNANCY ☐ YES ☐ NO | 9. COMPENSATION CASE ☐ YES ☐ NO | 10. WHEN, IN YOUR OPINION, DID PATIENT FIRST BECOME AWARE OF SOME SYMPTOM OF THIS CONDITION?

SURGICAL OR OBSTETRICAL PROCEDURES (DESCRIBE)

IF HOSPITALIZED, NAME AND ADDRESS OF HOSPITAL | 13. DATE ADMITTED | 14. DATE DISCHARGED

NAME AND ADDRESS OF OTHER PHYSICIANS WHO HAVE TREATED PATIENT FOR THIS ILLNESS OR INJURY

MPLETE IF PATIENT HAS INDICATED LOSS OF TIME BENEFITS

AUTHORIZATION TO PAY PHYSICIAN

TOTAL DISABILITY:

FROM _____ TO _____

PARTIAL DISABILITY:

FROM _____ TO _____

I HEREBY AUTHORIZE PAYMENT DIRECTLY TO THE ATTENDING PHYSICIAN FOR THIS ILLNESS OR INJURY, OF THE PHYSICIAN'S OR SURGEON'S BENEFITS OTHERWISE PAYABLE TO ME, BUT NOT TO EXCEED MY IN- DEBTEDNESS TO SAID PHYSICIAN. I UNDERSTAND I AM FINANCIALLY RESPONSIBLE TO THE PHYSICIAN FOR CHARGES NOT COVERED BY THIS ASSIGNMENT.

DATE _____ SIGNED _____
(INSURED)

☐ IS

THE HOSPITAL ☐ IS NOT AUTHORIZED TO FURNISH, WITH THE INSURED'S CONSENT, ANY INFORMATION REGARDING THIS CLAIM, REQUESTED BY THE _____ INSURANCE COMPANY.

>NED_____ | DATE_____
PHYSICIAN | DEGREE

CIAL SECURITY NO.
EMPLOYER I.D. NO._____ ADDRESS_____
STREET | CITY AND STATE | ZIP CODE

> NOTE TO PHYSICIAN: PLEASE SUBMIT YOUR ITEMIZED STATEMENT FOR THIS CLAIM. OKLAHOMA PHYSICIANS MAY USE OSMA FORM 102.

INSURED'S STATEMENT

TO BE COMPLETED PERSONALLY BY THE INSURED.
YOUR DOCTOR OR HOSPITAL IS NOT RESPONSIBLE FOR COMPLETION

.ICY NO_____ | CLAIM NO._____

ME | AGE | ADDRESS

F ACCIDENT: GIVE DATE | DESCRIBE HOW AND WHERE IT HAPPENED.

F SICKNESS: GIVE NATURE OF COMPLAINTS

>ATE YOU FIRST NOTICED SYMPTOMS OR REALIZED YOU WERE GETTING SICK | 4. DATE FIRST SAW A DOCTOR

HAVE YOU HAD SYMPTOMS OR TREATMENT FOR THIS SICKNESS BEFORE | 6. WHEN?

MEDICAL TREATMENT RECEIVED DURING LAST TWO YEARS

(SICKNESS) | (DOCTOR) | (YEAR)
ARE YOU MAKING CLAIM FOR LOSS OF TIME? ☐ YES ☐ NO

IF "YES": DATE FIRST STOPPED WORK: | FIRST DATE RETURNED TO WORK:

AUTHORIZATION   Reserve National Insurance Company
OKLAHOMA CITY, OKLAHOMA

I HEREBY AUTHORIZE ANY HOSPITAL OR PHYSICIAN TO FURNISH TO THE _____ INSURANCE MPANY OR ITS REPRESENTATIVE OR PERMIT SAID INSURANCE COMPANY OR ITS REPRESENTATIVE TO REVIEW ANY INFORMATION REQUESTED TH RESPECT TO ANY ILLNESS OR ACCIDENT, MEDICAL HISTORY OR COPIES OF HOSPITAL AND MEDICAL RECORDS. A PHOTOSTATIC COPY OF S AUTHORIZATION SHALL BE CONSIDERED AS VALID AS THE ORIGINAL. I DECLARE THE ABOVE ANSWERS AND STATEMENTS ARE TRUE AND RRECT TO THE BEST OF MY KNOWLEDGE AND BELIEF.

>TE _____ SIGNED: _____
INSURED

RM CL-18

**STANDARD LIFE & ACCIDENT INSURANCE COMPANY
OF CALIFORNIA**
5348 University Ave., San Diego, CA 92101

Complete the Comb-1 form and include the following as additional information. Use the question numbers shown so the company will know which of its questions you're answering. Be sure to provide an answer to every question, even if it's "No" or "None."

1a. If fracture or dislocation, describe nature and location.

4.   Give dates of other medical treatment, if any, during the past three years.

5.   Is patient still under your care for this condition? If "No," give date your services terminated.

6b. How long was or will patient be partially disabled?

STANDARD LIFE AND ACCIDENT INSURANCE COMPANY OF CALIFORNIA

ATTENDING PHYSICIAN'S STATEMENT—HEALTH INSURANCE CLAIM

ACCIDENT OR SICKNESS

ll Questions Must Be Answered

PATIENT'S NAME AND ADDRESS	AGE

1. (A) Diagnosis and Concurrent Conditions (If fracture or dislocation, describe nature and location.)

   (B) Is condition due to injury or sickness arising out of patient's employment? If "YES", explain.   Yes ☐   No ☐

2. (A) When did symptoms first appear or accident happen?   Date_____, 19___

   (B) When did patient first consult you for this condition?   Date_____, 19___

   (C) Has patient ever had same or similar condition? If "YES" state when and describe.   Yes ☐   No ☐

3. Nature of surgical procedure (describe fully).   Date performed_____, 19___

4. Give dates of other medical treatment, if any, during the past three years.

5. Is patient still under your care for this condition? If "NO" give date your services terminated.   Yes ☐   No ☐

   Date_____, 19___

6. (A) In your opinion, how long was or will the patient be continuously totally disabled and unable to work?   From_____, 19___   Thru_____, 19___

   (B) How long was or will patient be partially disabled?   From_____, 19___   Thru_____, 19___

DATE	SIGNATURE (ATTENDING PHYSICIAN)	DEGREE	TELEPHONE
STREET ADDRESS	CITY	STATE	ZIP CODE

EMPLOYER'S STATEMENT

INSURED CEASED WORK_____ A.M. ☐   P.M. ☐   because of accident ☐   sickness ☐
Date   Hour

If accident, was Insured injured while working?   Yes ☐   No ☐

Has Insured returned to work?   Yes ☐   No ☐   If yes, date returned_____, 19___

Insured occupational duties_____

Date_____   Signed_____

Employer   Employer's Title

Street Address   City   State   Telephone

UNITED FIDELITY LIFE INSURANCE COMPANY
1025 Elm St., Dallas, TX 75202

Complete the Comb-1 form and include the following as additional information. Use the question numbers shown so the company will know which of its questions you're answering. Be sure to provide an answer to every question, even if it's "No" or "None."

2. How long have you been the patient's doctor?

6. In your opinion, when did the basic cause of this condition originate?

7. Did you order hospital confinement for this patient?

9. What other physicians have treated this patient in the past?

10. Has patient any chronic or constitutional disease or physical defect? Give details.

12. To what other companies have you reported this claim?

L Questions MUST be answered

CLAIMANT'S STATEMENT FOR HOSPITAL AND/OR SURGICAL BENEFITS
(To be personally completed by the Insured)

Insured s Name .... Age .... Sex .... Policy # .. ..

If claim is made for a dependent covered by policy, answer following:

Name of dependent .... Age .... Relationship ....

What was the nature of the illness or injury? ....

(a) If injury, date it happened? .... (b) How did it happen? ....

....

On what date were symptoms of illness first noticed? ....

Name of first physician consulted? .... Date consulted? ....

When previously troubled with this or a similar condition? .. ..

What other medical or surgical treatment has been received during the past five years? (Give dates, nature of illnesses, or injuries, and names and addresses of attending physicians) ....

....

What other insurance do you have? ....

(accident, disability, hospital, or medical expense)

....

(Name of Company)

Have you, or do you intend to, present a claim for Workmen's Compensation arising out of this disability? Yes _____ No _____

I declare the foregoing answers and statements to be true and correct and I agree that if any are untrue, all rights under my policy shall be void. I hereby authorize any physician or hospital who has treated or attended me to furnish the UNITED FIDELITY LIFE INSURANCE COMPANY, or its representative, any information requested.

ed this .... day of .... 19 .... Signed ....

eet .... City .... State ....

ATTENDING PHYSICIAN'S REPORT

Patient's Name .... Age ....

How long have you been Patient's doctor? ....

On what date did you first attend Patient for this condition? ....

Describe in full the illness or injury with complete diagnosis? ....

....

....

(a) Contributing cause or conditions? ....

Has the Patient previously suffered from the same or similar condition? ....

In your opinion, when did the basic cause of this disability originate? ....

Did you order hospital confinement of the patient? ....

What surgical procedures were carried out? (Name each operation) ....

(a) Date of operation? ....

(b) What charge was made? ....

What other physicians have treated Patient in the past? ....

Has Patient any chronic or constitutional disease or physical defect? (give details) ....

On what dates did you personally visit the patient: At Office ....

At Hospital ....

At Home ....

To what other companies have you reported this claim? ....

Is condition due to injury or sickness arising out of patient's employment?..

hospital is hereby authorized to furnish, with the insured's consent, any information requested

e .... 19............ Signed...

IRS No........ ....

e to Attending Physician: Office Address..

Please indicate charges for hospital visits or attach
nized statement.   City...

- 109

WORKMEN'S BENEFIT FUND OF THE U.S.A.
714 Seneca Ave., Brooklyn, NY 11227

Complete the Comb-1 form and include the following as additional information. Use the question numbers shown so the company will know which of its questions you're answering. Be sure to provide an answer to every question, even if it's "No" or "None."

3. Name of hospital where you attended patient?

4. Please state how much of your total fee is due you or already paid by:
    - Patient or his family $
    - Blue Shield $
    - Medicare $
    - Other insurance (identify) $
                   TOTAL $

8. Was any mental or nervous disease or deficiency present?

FOUNDED 1884

WORKMEN'S BENEFIT FUND
OF THE UNITED STATES OF AMERICA
714 Seneca Ave., Brooklyn, N.Y. 11227

Cert. No._____
(HS-66)

ATTENDING PHYSICIAN'S STATEMENT
(For either Surgical or Medical Benefit, whichever is applicable) ·

Date of
1. Patient's Name (please PRINT): - - - - - - - - - - - - - Birth:- - - - -

   Address: -
2. Nature of sickness or injury: -
3. Hospital where attended: -
4. Kind of operation or treatment (if operation, state date): - - - - - -
   -

   State total fee for above service, no matter BY WHOM PAID or payable

   $ - - - - -

   Please state how much of above sum is due you from, or paid by:

   ◯ Patient or his family $- - - - -)
   ◯ Blue Shield $- - - - -⟩
   ◯ Medicare $- - - - -⟩
   ◯ Other Insurance or Coverage (identify) $- - - - -⟩ Total:
                                              $ _____

   -
5. (To be completed if treated medically at hospital)
   Exact dates of hospital visits: - - - - - - - - - - - - - - - - - - -
   -
   Total number of visits: - - - - Charge per visit: $ - - - - -
6. Did the procedure bear any relationship to co-existing pregnancy or
   childbirth? ◯ Yes   ◯ No
   If yes, state details: -
7. Is this a Workmen's Compensation case? ◯ Yes   ◯ No
8. Was any mental or nervous disease or deficiency present? ◯ Yes ◯ No
9. When were symptoms of present condition first noted? - - - - - - - - --
0. Remarks: -

Date: Doctor's address
   - - - - - -   Stamp:
                                                Signature

Index